Tips for the Residency Match

✓ TIPS FOR THE

RESIDENCY MATCH

What Residency Directors Are Really Looking For

Edited by

Justin W. Kung, MD
Associate Program Director, Radiology
Assistant Professor of Radiology
Beth Israel Deaconess Medical Center
Harvard Medical School
Boston, MA, USA

Priscilla J. Slanetz, MD, MPH
Program Director, Radiology
Associate Professor of Radiology
Beth Israel Deaconess Medical Center
Harvard Medical School
Boston, MA, USA

Pauline M. Bishop, MD
Clinical Fellow in Interventional Radiology
Beth Israel Deaconess Medical Center
Harvard Medical School
Boston, MA, USA

Ronald L. Eisenberg, MD, JD
Associate Program Director, Radiology
Professor of Radiology
Beth Israel Deaconess Medical Center
Harvard Medical School
Boston, MA, USA

WILEY Blackwell

Registered Office
John Wiley & Sons Ltd, The Atrium, Southern Gate, Chichester, West Sussex, PO19 8SQ, UK

Editorial Offices
350 Main Street, Malden, MA 02148-5020, USA
9600 Garsington Road, Oxford, OX4 2DQ, UK
The Atrium, Southern Gate, Chichester, West Sussex, PO19 8SQ, UK

For details of our global editorial offices, for customer services, and for information about how to apply for permission to reuse the copyright material in this book please see our website at www.wiley.com/wiley-blackwell.

The right of Justin W. Kung, Pauline M. Bishop, Priscilla J. Slanetz and Ronald L. Eisenberg to be identified as the authors of the editorial material in this work has been asserted in accordance with the UK Copyright, Designs and Patents Act 1988.

Library of Congress Cataloging-in-Publication Data

Tips for the residency match : what residency directors are really looking for / edited by Justin W. Kung, Pauline M. Bishop, Priscilla J. Slanetz, Ronald L. Eisenberg.
       p. ; cm.
  Includes bibliographic references and index.
  ISBN 978-1-118-86093-9 (pbk.)
  I. Kung, Justin W., editor. II. Bishop, Pauline M., editor. III. Slanetz, Priscilla J., editor. IV. Eisenberg, Ronald L., editor.
  [DNLM: 1. Internship and Residency–United States. 2. Career Choice–United States. 3. Professional
Competence–United States. 4. Students, Medical–United States. 5. Vocational Guidance–United States. W 20]
  R840
  610.71'55–dc23
                              2014037411

A catalogue record for this book is available from the British Library.

Set in 10.5/14 Adobe Garamond Pro by Aptara, Inc., New Delhi, India
Printed and bound in Singapore by Markono Print Media Pte Ltd

1   2015

This book is dedicated to our families for their understanding and support:
To the three girls in my life: Adrienne, Evelyn, and Ava   J.W.K.
For my daughter, Kaylie, and my husband, Kristoffer   P.M.B.
To Raja, Robert, Natalie, and Helen   P.J.S.
To Zina, Avlana, and Cherina   R.L.E.

Contents

Contributors

Faculty

Rina Bloch, MD
Associate Professor
Program Director, Physical Medicine and Rehabilitation
Tufts University School of Medicine
Boston, MA, USA

Robert P. Bonacci, MD
Assistant Professor
Program Director, Family Medicine
The Mayo Clinic
Rochester, MN, USA

Anthony Chang, MD
Associate Professor
Associate Program Director, Pathology
Pritzker School of Medicine
University of Chicago
Chicago, IL, USA

David Chong, MD
Assistant Professor
Associate Program Director, Internal Medicine
Columbia University College of Physicians and Surgeons
New York, NY, USA

Kenneth B. Christopher, MD
Instructor in Medicine
Assistant Program Director, Internal Medicine

Brigham and Women's Hospital
Harvard Medical School
Boston, MA, USA

George S. M. Dyer, MD
Assistant Professor
Program Director, Orthopedic Surgery
Harvard Combined Orthopaedic Residency Program
Harvard Medical School
Boston, MA, USA

Benjamin L. Judson, MD
Assistant Professor
Associate Program Director, Otolaryngology
Yale School of Medicine
New Haven, CT, USA

William Krauss, MD
Professor
Program Director, Neurosurgery
The Mayo Clinic
Rochester, MN, USA

Jennifer L. Kurth, DO
Assistant Professor
Northwestern University Feinberg School of Medicine
Chicago, IL, USA
Former Program Director, Psychiatry
Loyola University Medical Center
Chicago, IL, USA

Yvette LaCoursiere, MD
Associate Clinical Professor
Program Director, Obstetrics and
Gynecology
UCSD School of Medicine
San Diego, CA, USA

James N. Lau, MD
Clinical Associate Professor
Associate Program Director, Surgery
Stanford University School of Medicine
Stanford, CA, USA

Zachary N. London, MD
Associate Professor
Program Director, Neurology
University of Michigan Medical School
Ann Arbor, MI, USA

Suzanne Long, MD
Assistant Professor
Program Director, Radiology
Thomas Jefferson University Hospital
Jefferson Medical College
Philadelphia, PA, USA

Elias M. Michaelides, MD
Assistant Professor
Program Director, Otolaryngology
Yale School of Medicine
New Haven, CT, USA

Heather McPhillips, MD, MPH
Professor
Program Director, Pediatrics
University of Washington School of
Medicine and Seattle Children's
Hospital
Seattle, WA, USA

Qi Cui Ott, MD
Instructor
Associate Program Director, Anesthesia
Beth Israel Deaconess Medical Center
Harvard Medical School
Boston, MA, USA

Andrew C. Peterson, MD, FACS
Associate Professor
Program Director, Urology
Duke University Medical Center
Durham, NC, USA

Rachel Reynolds, MD
Assistant Professor
Program Director, Dermatology
Harvard Combined Dermatology
Residency Training Program
Harvard Medical School
Boston, MA, USA

Carlo L. Rosen, MD
Associate Professor
Program Director, Emergency
Medicine
Associate Director, Graduate Medical
Education
Beth Israel Deaconess Medical Center
Harvard Medical School
Boston, MA, USA

Pierre Saadeh, MD
Assistant Professor
Program Director, Plastic Surgery
New York University School of
Medicine
New York, NY, USA

Paul Tapino, MD
Associate Professor
Program Director, Ophthalmology
Scheie Eye Institute
Perelman School of Medicine
University of Pennsylvania Medical School
Philadelphia, PA, USA

Stephanie Terezakis, MD
Assistant Professor
Program Director, Radiation Oncology
John Hopkins University School of
Medicine
Baltimore, MD, USA

Carrie D. Tibbles, MD
Assistant Professor
Director Graduate Medical Education
Beth Israel Deaconess Medical Center
Harvard Medical School
Boston, MA, USA

Jim S. Wu, MD
Assistant Professor
Former Program Director, Radiology
Beth Israel Deaconess Medical Center
Harvard Medical School
Boston, MA, USA

Residents

Shushmita M. Ahmed, MD
Resident, General Surgery
Stanford University School of Medicine
Stanford, CA, USA

Sara Alcorn, MD, MPH
Resident, Radiation Oncology
John Hopkins University School of
Medicine
Baltimore, MD, USA

Jason S. Barr, MD
Resident, Plastic Surgery
New York University School of Medicine
New York, NY, USA

Laura Chen, MD
Resident, Pediatrics
University of Washington School of Medicine and
Seattle Children's Hospital
Seattle, WA, USA

Steven T. Chen, MD, MPH
Resident, Dermatology
Harvard Combined Dermatology Residency
Training Program
Harvard Medical School
Boston, MA, USA

Bonnie Choy, MD
Resident, Pathology
Pritzker School of Medicine
University of Chicago
Chicago, IL, USA

Amy Downing, MD
Resident, Pediatrics
University of Washington School of Medicine and
Seattle Children's Hospital
Seattle, WA, USA

Kathleen Dunn, MD
Resident, Obstetrics and Gynecology
UCSD School of Medicine
San Diego, CA, USA

Kian Eftekhari, MD
Resident, Ophthalmology
Scheie Eye Institute
Perelman School of Medicine
University of Pennsylvania Medical
School
Philadelphia, PA, USA

Jacob Erickson, DO
Instructor
Resident, Family Medicine
The Mayo Clinic
Rochester, MN, USA

Shannon Fitzgerald, MD
Medical Student
Harvard Medical School
Boston, MA, USA

Michael Granieri, MD
Resident, Urology
Duke University Medical Center
Durham, NC, USA

Elena B. Hawryluk, MD, PhD
Resident, Dermatology
Harvard Combined Dermatology Residency
Training Program
Harvard Medical School
Boston, MA, USA

Joseph Kapurch, MD
Resident, Neurosurgery
The Mayo Clinic
Rochester, MN, USA

Mary Lally, BMBCh
Resident, Family Medicine
The Mayo Clinic
Rochester, MN, USA

Christine Miller, MD
Resident, Obstetrics and
Gynecology
UCSD School of Medicine
San Diego, CA, USA

Vinod E. Nambudiri, MD, MBA
Resident, Dermatology
Harvard Combined Dermatology Residency
Training Program
Harvard Medical School
Boston, MA, USA

Boris Paskhover, MD
Resident, Otolaryngology
Yale School of Medicine
New Haven CT, USA

Michaela Restivo, MD
Resident, Internal Medicine
Columbia University College of Physicians
and Surgeons
New York, NY, USA

Samir Shah, MD
Resident, Radiology
Beth Israel Deaconess Medical Center
Harvard Medical School
Boston, MA, USA

Amanda Trotter, MD
Resident, Radiology
Beth Israel Deaconess Medical
Center
Harvard Medical School
Boston, MA, USA

Natalie Wheeler, MD, JD
Resident, Neurology
University of Michigan Medical School
Ann Arbor, MI, USAThe Mayo Clinic
Rochester, MN, USA

Preface

Every year, thousands of medical students from the United States and abroad apply for residency positions through the Match. The application process can be chaotic, as students struggle to choose a future career path based upon limited exposure while at the same time trying to juggle their clinical responsibilities. In this book, we attempt to simplify and summarize the Match process. In Chapter 1: *The Match Alphabet Soup*, we break down the Match, giving readers insight into the history behind it, the technical intricacies of the match process, and the strategy behind the match algorithm. There are multiple organizations and acronyms associated with the Match, including the NRMP, ERAS, ECFMG, and SOAP, and we explain how they all have a role in the Match process.

Preparation is key. In reality, students are preparing for the Match from the first day they enter medical school and are wrestling with the very important decision of specialty selection. Students need to be aware of specific steps that they must take in medical school in order to position themselves for a great match. We highlight those steps which should be taken, beginning in the first year of medical school right up to the Match. We also discuss the very difficult choice of specialty selection, which is a complicated interplay of student preference and realistic expectations. A match in Dermatology and Plastic Surgery may not be attainable by every applicant. However, through a process of **S**elf-assessment, **E**xploration, **L**ikelihood, and **F**allback (**SELF**), every student can select a specialty best suited towards his/her individual talents.

What exactly is a Program Director looking for in your application? How important are pre-interview dinners? There are multiple **Insider Tips** offered throughout this book based upon years of experience in the residency selection process. We offer a unique look into the Match through the eyes of a Program Director. What is the selection process really like? We detail this in Chapter 5: *The Selection Process – Theirs*. We also offer a detailed look at every specialty, including the information you always wanted to know but were afraid to ask, such as salary and lifestyle. These individual specialty-specific chapters are written by some of the nation's top Program Directors and their residents from institutions including Harvard, Yale, John Hopkins, Duke, Columbia, Stanford, UCSD, Mayo Clinic, and many more. Specialty specific insights are provided by leaders in fields ranging from Neurosurgery to Psychiatry.

Finally, International Medical Graduates (IMGs) play a crucial role in providing healthcare in the United States, but the path to the Match can be more arduous. We offer specific advice important to IMGs in areas including USLME preparation, research fellowships, and specialty selection.

We hope that you enjoy and profit from this book.

Acknowledgements

This book would not have been possible without the support of many people, and we wish to express our thanks and appreciation to all of them.

- The medical students and residents with whom we have had the privilege of working and training
- The countless numbers of Harvard Medical Students who have read portions of this book and offered us suggestions
- Mei Liang, Director of Research at the National Resident Matching Program (NRMP®), for thoughtful advice and encouragement
- Dr. Ammar Sarwar and Dr. Robert Kung for their very helpful comments
- Clotell Forde for her assistance in preparing the manuscript
- Our families, for their understanding, encouragement, and support

Disclaimer

The information contained in this book is strictly for informational purposes. The editors and authors of this book have used their best efforts in preparing this book, but make no representations or warranties with respect to the accuracy, applicability, fitness, or completeness of the information contained in this book. The information in this book is provided "as-is" and without warranty. The editors and authors shall not be liable to any party (including, without limitation, the reader) for any direct, indirect, special, punitive, consequential, or other damages arising out of or relating to, in both cases directly or indirectly, from the use of the information in this book. Names and specific facts used in examples and anecdotes have been altered to protect the identity of individuals. Information regarding the subject matter of this book may change rapidly and readers are solely responsible for checking program application deadlines, fees, dates, or any other requirements.

About the Editors

Justin W. Kung is an Assistant Professor of Radiology at Harvard Medical School and a radiologist at the Beth Israel Deaconess Medical Center in Boston. He serves as an Associate Residency Director and has specific interests in medical student education.

Pauline M. Bishop is an Interventional Radiology Fellow and former Radiology resident at Beth Israel Deaconess Medical Center in Boston.

Priscilla J. Slanetz is an Associate Professor of Radiology at Harvard Medical School and a radiologist at the Beth Israel Deaconess Medical Center in Boston, where she is the Residency Director. A Fellow of the American College of Radiology, she holds an MPH in Health Policy and Management from the Harvard School of Public Health.

Ronald L. Eisenberg is Professor of Radiology at Harvard Medical School and a radiologist at the Beth Israel Deaconess Medical Center in Boston. An Associate Residency Director, he is the author of more than 20 books in radiology. A Fellow of the American College of Radiology, Dr. Eisenberg is also a non-practising lawyer and author of *Radiology and the Law: Malpractice and Other Issues* (Springer).

Introduction

Congratulations! If you are purchasing this book, you are either nearing the end of medical school and crossing a major hurdle in your training, or you are in your preclinical years and planning ahead for residency application. Both possibilities deserve praise.

Besides passing your medical school classes and boards (a feat unto itself), you have two incredibly important decisions to make: choosing a specialty and then a residency. These decisions are extremely nerve-racking for a medical student. You are only just starting to feel comfortable in your book-based knowledge and now, with very little information about actual clinical practice, you are compelled to choose a career path and the training program that will get you started on it. It is a decision that requires truthful introspection about both your professional and equally important personal goals. No doubt, your energies have been so fixated on short-term objectives, such as getting good grades on exams, that you have had little time to consider the bigger picture. What sort of life do you actually want? A specialty choice will play a large role in achieving that life. Once you have narrowed down the field to one or two potential specialties, it is time to take another honest look at your academic performance. Can you actually get a residency position in your desired specialty?

The 2013 National Residency Matching Program® (NRMP®) results revealed that it was the most competitive year to date, with a total of 40 335 registrants and 34 355 active applicants submitting applications for 29 171 positions, 26 392 of which were available at the first postgraduate year (PGY-1) level (Figure I.1). This represents a sharp increase compared with the 38 377 registrants in 2012, an upsurge due largely to several new US allopathic medical schools graduating their first classes, adding up to nearly 1000 new registrants. The increase was also largely affected by approximately 800 more US citizens studying abroad (US International Medical Graduate (IMGs)) and hoping to return to the United States for their residency education, not to mention 740 more non-US citizen IMG applicants in 2013 compared with 2012 [1]. Even after discounting those initial registrants who eventually withdrew from consideration, or, as the NRMP would put it, were no longer "active", there were only 0.77 available PGY-1 residency positions per active applicant! Not only has the Match become increasingly competitive as a whole, but as the cost of medical education rises, more and more graduating medical students are forced to consider future income as a major factor in specialty selection. This causes certain subspecialty residency programs to be disproportionately competitive.

As competition for residency increases without a relative increase in residency positions, now more than ever it is important to understand what a Program Director is looking for in an applicant. The primary and contributing authors of this book represent several combined decades of Program Director experience, which has demonstrated that graduating medical students undervalue their worth by emphasizing the wrong facets of their applications. We

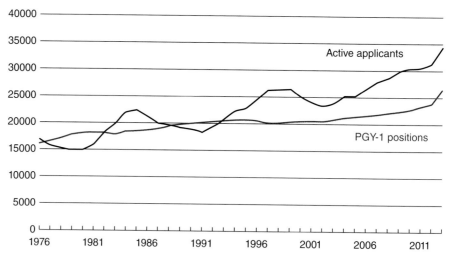

Figure I.1 Active applicants versus PGY-1 positions, 1976–2013. *Source:* Adapted with permission from [1].

will aim to bridge the gap between medical students' perceptions of a solid application and the perceptions of residency Program Directors.

We will teach you how to build a strong application from the moment you start medical school right up to Match Day, while at the same time investigating the specialties so you can find the right fit for you. Specialty selection is a daunting process; we will walk you through the steps involved and factors to consider. In addition, in Chapter 3: *The Specialties – Program Directors' Perspectives*, we provide more detailed specialty-specific information, provided by Program Directors of some of the top residency programs in the country, ranging from competitiveness of the application process to a frank discussion of salary and lifestyle expectations after residency.

Once you have decided on a specialty, it is time to dive into the residency Match. We will discuss the particulars of the application process, including a clear explanation of the complex matching algorithm as well as recent updates in the "All In Policy" and the Supplemental Offer and Acceptance Program® (SOAP®), and explain how these may affect your rank order list (ROL). Furthermore, we will teach you how to highlight key components of your curriculum vitae and personal statement in order to increase your chances of being invited for an interview and how to excel on interview day once it arrives. Many programs meet shortly, if not immediately, after each applicant interview session to plan their ROL. We reveal how these decisions are made; you may be surprised by how subjective the evaluations are. However, with the help of this book, you can use those idiosyncrasies to your advantage.

Insider Tips from highly regarded residency Program Directors are peppered throughout this book. Here are just a sample of tips that are generally true across all subspecialties. Each will be discussed in more detail in their dedicated chapters.

Insider Tip 1: Perceived commitment and understanding of a specialty is one of the most important factors that Program Directors use in choosing a residency applicant.

Insider Tip 2: Begin to think about how to set yourself apart on paper. An interesting application translates into an interesting interview, which is something every Program Director wants.

Insider Tip 3: Networking is essential at all levels of your medical career, from medical school through residency training all the way to the attending level.

Insider Tip 4: Consider doing away electives. They are a chance for both you and the program to scratch beneath the surface.

Insider Tip 5: Everything about interview day is important. But remember, though *Roget's Thesaurus* may disagree, when it comes to interview day, strange is not a synonym for interesting.

Insider Tip 6: Seek out an advocate on the selection committee. When everyone looks the same on paper, having even one person on the committee offer up an extra positive remark can make all the difference.

Insider Tip 7: Do not alter your ROL based on communication or lack of communication from residency programs after interview day is complete. Even if you send a communication expressing interest, do not expect to receive a response back from the program.

Insider Tip 8: Seek letters of recommendation both from physicians respected in the field and those who know you well. Ideally, they are the same person. If not, try to satisfy both factors when choosing letter writers.

Insider Tip 9: Do not disregard your extracurricular activities when completing your application. They help paint a picture of you as a person. Your future attendings want to know and like the person who is waking them up in the middle of the night.

Insider Tip 10: Be polite throughout the entire process. The person you cutoff driving into the hospital parking garage that morning may be one of interviewers later that day (true story!).

Our goal is that by the end of this book, you will be able to make an educated decision about a career choice, and then work towards that choice with a thorough understanding of the match process and a realistic appreciation of your residency competitiveness.

Reference

1. NRMP (2013) *Results and Data: 2013 Main Residency Match®*. National Resident Matching Program: Washington, DC.

1: The Match Alphabet Soup

The term "*the* Match" may have led you to believe that there is but one residency matching program, when in actuality there are several. However, the National Residency Matching Program (NRMP®) is the program used by the vast majority of medical school seniors, so "the Match" refers to it unless otherwise specified. In brief, the other matching systems include the Military Match, the SF Match (San Francisco Matching Program), the Urology Match, and the American Osteopathic Association (AOA) Match. The SF Match (www.SFmatch.org) is specifically for Ophthalmology, Neurotology, and some Plastic Surgery programs. However, all of these specialties require completion of some preliminary residency training that is likely arranged through participation in the traditional NRMP. Of note, while Child Neurology and Neurotology allow completion of both matching processes simultaneously, those Plastic Surgery programs utilizing the SF Match require completion of 3–4 years of general surgical residency before applying to Plastic Surgery. Urology also has a separate matching program (Urology Residency Matching Program (URMP); www.auanet.org). The URMP has an earlier timeline (January) than the NRMP (March), an important fact when considering backup specialty applications. The URMP may still receive its applications through the Electronic Residency Application Services (ERAS®), or via universal applications, or by applications created by the programs themselves. Finally, there is a separate AOA-sponsored match (www.osteopathic.org) called the National Matching Service (NMS) for graduates of osteopathic medical schools (DOs as opposed to allopathic medical school graduates, MDs) which occurs in February. Note that DOs may apply to American College of Graduate Medical Education (ACGME)-approved residency and fellowship programs via the NRMP, though not vice versa. However, given (perceived) differences in medical training, as well as separate board examinations (DOs take the Comprehensive Osteopathic Medical Licensing Examination of the United States (COMLEX-USA®), while MDs take the United States Medical Licensing Examination® (USMLE®)), DO graduates have traditionally had difficulty in successfully matching to ACGME programs, particularly in Surgery (see Chapter 4: *Path to the Match* and Chapter 5: *The Selection Process – Theirs*). Be mindful that an applicant who receives a spot through the earlier AOA-NMS Match is automatically withdrawn from the NRMP.

A confusing factor in the application process is the relationship between NRMP and ERAS (and why you will need to register and pay fees to both organizations). The NRMP's Main Residency Match® is a private, non-profit, non-governmental organization created in 1952 to help match medical school students with residency programs. It is sponsored in part by the American Board of Medical Specialties (ABMS), the American Medical Association (AMA), and the Association of American Medical Colleges (AAMC). The NRMP was born in response to a shortage of residency program graduates, resulting in severe competition among hospitals to hire new interns [1, 2]. In the hope of enticing desirable candidates, hospitals began to make offers as early as 2 years before graduation. Conversely, students stalled acceptance as long as possible while waiting for a better offer. As you can imagine, it was an incredibly dysfunctional process, and both parties cried out for a more transparent and efficient system.

The Main Residency Match is managed through the NRMP's Registration, Ranking, and Results (R3®) system, which provides a consistent and objective path by which all participants, both residency programs and applicants, must abide. The system prevents programs from offering residency positions with the attached threat of an expiration date, thus eliminating the pressure students feel to accept their first offer rather than their first choice. It is essentially a computer following a programmed algorithm that maximizes the preferences of both applicants and residency programs by "matching" the two based on their rank order lists (ROLs). Secondarily, an applicant may acquire an unfilled position as part of the Match Week Supplemental Offer and Acceptance Program (SOAP®). All participants in the Match are expected to proceed in an ethical and professional manner, so that medical students can consider all prospective programs without external pressure. As an applicant, you will electronically sign a participation agreement saying that you will abide by the standards and results of the Match. This process has taken another step in the direction of protecting the rights of the applicant with the 2013 implementation of the NRMP's "All In Policy," which requires participating programs to include "all" or "none" of their positions in the match [3]. Prior to this change, programs could offer "pre-matches" to independent applicants – a group which includes all applicants except US senior allopathic medical students. International Medical Graduates (IMGs) (both US citizens and not) receiving a pre-match offer considered it a safe bet and never participated in the match, which may have limited their potential for the ideal fit. An interesting side-effect of this new policy is that there appears to be many more residency positions offered in 2013 than in the past. However, a majority of these are due to residency spots previously filled by pre-match offers.

It is important to remember that the NRMP is *not* an application service. It is purely a matching service, to which you must register and pay separately ($65 for the first 20 programs and $30 for each additional program as of 2014). Candidates must apply directly to the residency programs. However, the majority of programs (including AOA programs) have standardized this process by requiring that students submit applications to them via ERAS, which electronically (via the internet-based "PostOffice") transmits your application to these programs. ERAS is basically a digital manila folder with your photograph, personal statement, Medical School Performance Evaluation (MSPE, the former "Dean's letter"), letters of recommendation (LoRs), medical school transcripts, board scores (USMLE or COMLEX), and extracurricular activities. While ERAS has centralized all the components of the application, the applicant is still responsible for knowing the deadlines and providing any additional material requested by individual programs. This information is usually readily available on a residency program's website. As an alternative, the information can be quickly obtained by contacting the residency program coordinator. The ERAS fee schedule is based on the number of programs to which you apply. The ERAS fee breakdown in 2014 was:

- First 10 programs: $95
- Programs 11–20: $10 each
- Programs 21–30: $16 each
- Programs ≥ 31: $26 each

Depending on the competitiveness of the specialty, you may have to apply to a few dozen programs. In 2013, the average number of programs to which a successfully matched applicant applied reached a whopping 29 programs, whereas those who failed to match applied to an average of 50 programs [4].

Let us do the math:

Total fees:
NRMP fees ($65 + $30 per program if >20 programs ranked) + ERAS fees + boards transcript release fee (COMLEX/USMLE; cost $70)

20 programs:
ERAS fees: $95 + (10 programs × $10) = $195
NRMP fees: $65
Board transcript release fee = $70
Total fees = $330

30 programs:
ERAS fees: $95 + (10 programs × $10) + (10 programs × $16) = $355
NRMP fees: $65 + (10 additional programs × $30 per program) = $365
Board transcript release fee = $70
Total fees = $790

Of course, this does not include the cost associated with interviews, primarily travel expenses. Therefore, although casting a wider net obviously increases your chances of matching, for most people the cost (and allowed time off for interviews) is prohibitive. This is one of the many reasons it is important to understand how competitive a candidate you are in the eyes of Program Directors.

> **Insider Tip:** Budget your time and application expenses wisely. Residencies can begin to download applications on September 15 as soon as you pay the registration fees. Many offer interviews before your application is even complete, which technically is not until your designated Dean's Office uploads your MSPE (on or after October 1).

If you are feeling a little lost in the alphabet soup of the application process, Figure 1.1 is a general overview that includes the more common abbreviations.

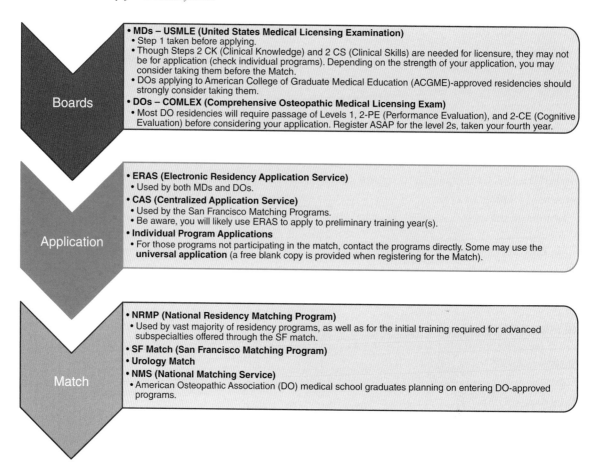

Figure 1.1 Residency application alphabet soup.

The Match Algorithm and the Secrets to Stable Marriage

The NRMP is essentially a clearinghouse of residency MD positions:

- **Categorical (C):** Entering during your first postgraduate year (PGY-1) and continuing there until completing your training for specialty certification, generally 3–5 years.
- **Preliminary (P):** 1 (or 2) year(s) of prerequisite training during PGY-1 (and PGY-2) prior to entry into advanced specialty programs. These can be further subdivided into Internal Medicine, Surgery, and Transitional Year programs (usually some combination of the former).
- **Advanced (A):** Specialty training that is often 3–4 years in length and begins after completion of 1–2 years of preliminary training (beginning PGY-2 or PGY-3).
- **Primary Care Categorical (M):** A small group of Medicine and Pediatrics programs offer this option.

- **Physician (R):** For physicians with prior graduate medical education applying for advanced training through the match.

Applicants interview at residency programs all over the country and then submit ROLs indicating their preference among the interviewed positions. The residency programs, in turn, submit their ROLs of the interviewed applicants in addition to the number of positions available. The NRMP processes these ROLs based on the applied algorithm and produces a "stable" match. Stable is defined by *not* creating a pair of matching agents (applicants and residency spots) who would mutually prefer to be matched to each other rather than adhere to the match produced by the clearinghouse.

Drs. Alvin E. Roth (Harvard University, Cambridge) and Lloyd S. Shapely (University of California, Los Angeles) were awarded the Nobel Prize in Economic Science in 2012 for developing the theory of stable allocations and the practice of market design through the combined efforts of Shapely's game theory study and Roth's recognition of the practical applications of the theory, including implementation during the NRMP Match process [5]. The work drew on the Gale–Shapely theory of "stable marriage," first explored in the 1960s. It explained how deferred acceptance of an offer of marriage could achieve stability and satisfaction of choice among mates [6]. In 1984, Dr. Roth pointed out that the success of the NRMP Match was based on its extrapolation of the stable marriage concept [6]. However, in the mid-1990s, residents began to lose confidence in the Match system, citing concerns that it favored the interests of residency programs over students. Thus, students began to try to "game the system" by submitting ROLs based on strategy rather than preference [7]. Realizing that lack of faith in the Match would inevitably lead to its collapse, in 1995 the NRMP commissioned the design of a new algorithm that would favor the applicants as much as possible. It also conducted an inquiry into the number of more-preferred versus less-preferred matches produced by the two methods and whether strategic behavior could affect the outcome using either algorithm [1].

Much of the 1990s controversy about the impartiality of the Match was in response to theoretical literature stating that the stable marriage principle has two basic versions in which one side, either the husband or the wife (the student or the residency program), makes offers that the other side can reject or hold to see if a better offer comes along. Basically, whose "Top 10 Spouses" (the husband or the wife's) or, as in our case, whose ROL (applicant or residency) should be the starting point? The older algorithm had been analyzed in a theoretical simple market and suggested that this contention may be correct; whose list was the starting point of the algorithm, residency-proposed list versus applicant-proposed list, may make a difference. However, the NRMP is not a simple market of only a husband and wife; there are at least four kinds of match variations beyond the basic categorical match [1]:

1. Couples seeking positions geographically near one another
2. Applicants seeking PGY-2 positions and, if successful, have supplemental lists to match them to their prerequisite PGY-1 spots
3. Residency programs with positions that revert to other programs if they remain unfilled
4. Programs that wish to fill an even number of positions if they cannot fill all their available positions (e.g., the residency has six available positions, but for a variety

First Round

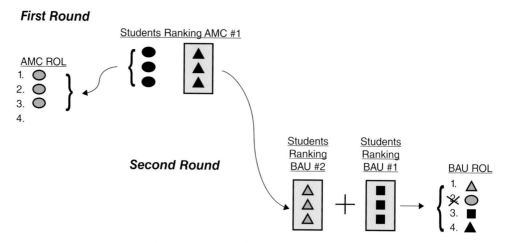

Figure 1.2 Hypothetical match process.

of reasons including ease of scheduling, will only accept four residents, even if five desirable residents are available for match)

Let us initially imagine that the Match *is* a simple market. Hypothetically, we have two residency programs. Amazing Medical Center (AMC), the first choice of most, and Better than Average University (BAU), which is less popular but still highly respectable. Both have three available residency positions. Imagine that the algorithm proceeds in separate static steps (Figure 1.2). In the first round, everyone wants to go to AMC. Once a population of students wanting to go to the same institution is defined, the top students in that pool, as determined by that program's ROL, will match there. In the second round, the remaining unmatched students who ranked AMC as #1 and BAU as #2 are now pooled with those students who ranked BAU #1. Of that pool, the top students as determined by BAU's ROL are matched. Note that the student BAU had ranked as a second choice had already matched at AMC, so BAU had to "go further down their ROL" in order to fill all three positions.

Although the process is presented as subsequent steps, in reality this is a dynamic process that is continuously adjusted every time a student is added to the pool. For instance, all three of the students ranking BAU #1 were initially tentatively matched there, but once the selection pool was redefined by the addition of students not matching to AMC, two of those (■) students were essentially bumped out of those spots by students who ranked BAU second but were preferred by the residency program. Hopefully, those students ranked more programs on their ROL and will still be in the running for the next computation.

> **Insider Tip:** Though it may be intuitive, scientific analysis has confirmed that the more programs you rank, the better your odds are of matching. Do not rely on promises of high rankings from your potential programs and mistakenly think you only need to submit a short ROL.

The 1995 analysis of the simple matching algorithm demonstrated that use of the old residency-proposed algorithm rather than one based on applicant-proposed matches led to a very small number of cases (0.1%) in which applicants would have matched to higher-ranked programs with the applicant-proposed match system [1]. Thus, the algorithm was changed to an applicant-centric method that (slightly) favors the student. The new algorithm was successfully incorporated beginning in 1998.

You may have noticed that creating stable matches based on the applicant ROL means that if a student prefers a program different from the one to which he/she matched, he/she must have applied to that program and been rejected. Therefore, the applicant-proposed version of the algorithm gives each student his/her most preferred position for which he/she was eligible. Therefore, in response to NRMP concerns of adjusting a ROL based on strategy rather than preference, two interesting facts were demonstrated. First, the high cost of multiple interviews incurred by both applicant and programs placed a practical limit on how many interviews were conducted, severely limiting the ability to employ strategy when composing a ROL. Second, the complex market of the NRMP closely approximated the simple theoretical stable marriage match and a simple applicant-proposed algorithm gave no opportunity for an applicant to improve his/her match by submitting a ROL that differed from his/her true preferences.

Insider Tip: No games! Rank your list based on your true preferences rather than which program you think will rank you higher. You may match further down your list, but you will match at the highest position that was actually available to you.

Adding couples who submit joint preferences into the equation makes generation of a stable match much more difficult. In some cases, there is no stable solution, meaning it is impossible to avoid creating unmatched pairs who would prefer each other to their actual match. Essentially, couples are tentatively matched individually and then reject the position, until they reach a point on their list where both applicants find their position acceptable. Unfortunately, couples are more likely to match worse together than had they applied individually. To better explain this point we will switch from a graphical representation of the match algorithm to a tabular one, similar to that provided on the NRMP "Run a Match" webpage [8], as the steps are more complex to consider with two paired applicants.

Imagine Diana and Frank are a Boston-based couple trying to couples match. Their top choices include AMC and Copacetic Community Hospital (CCH), both in New England, while BAU and Dime a Dozen Hospital (DDH) are a 4-hour drive south in New York. For the sake of simplicity, we will assume that a program's station in the alphabet is a measure of its overall popularity. Given these geographic considerations, with Diana being a strong candidate in a less competitive field, Diana and Frank rank the following possible matches at the top of their list:

	Diana	Frank
1	AMC	AMC
2	BAU	BAU
3	AMC	CCH
4	BAU	DDH
5	No match	BAU

However, they are competing with the following single applicants and their ROLs:

	Amy	Ben	Charlie	Elliot
1	AMC	AMC	AMC	AMC
2	BAU	BAU	BAU	BAU
3	CCH	DDH	CCH	CCH

Each potential program has two vacant spots and they have the following ROLs:

	AMC	BAU	CCH	DDH
1	Amy	Diana	Amy	Ben
2	Diana	Amy	Charlie	Amy
3	Ben	Charlie	Ben	Diana
4	Charlie	Frank	Frank	Frank
5		Ben	Elliot	

First Round

Applicant	ROL	Program status	Match result
Amy	1. AMC	Two open slots	Match (both parties picked the other as #1)
Ben	1. AMC	One open slot	Tentative match (other students are ranked higher)
Charlie	1. AMC	Ranks lower than current spot holders	No match
	2. BAU	Two open slots	Tentative match (other students are ranked higher)
Elliot	1. AMC	Ranks lower than current spot holders	No match
	2. CCH	Two open slots	Tentative match (other students are ranked higher)
Diana/ Frank	1. AMC/AMC	Though Diana was ranked higher than Ben, Frank was not ranked here so there is no match	
	2. BAU/BAU	One open slot; though Diana is ranked first here, Frank is not ranked higher than Charlie and thus unable to take the second spot so there is no match	
	3. AMC/CCH	CCH has one open slot and Frank is tentatively matched here and Diana bumps Ben from AMC	Tentative match, Diana at AMC and Frank at CCH

Second round, Ben was bumped from AMC by Diana, so we move to his second choice:

Second Round (Version 1)

Applicant	ROL	Program status	Match result
Ben	1. AMC	Spots now filled by Amy and Diana	
	2. BAU	One spot	Tentative match

Ben, matching as a single applicant and without the same geographical concerns as our couple, opted for the second most popular school, taking the as yet unfilled spot at BAU. This version was provided to show you how it is possible for all parties to come to a stable match. However, if Ben really wanted to stay in Boston and had chosen CCH as his second choice, he was ranked higher than Frank and would have bumped Frank and thus the entire pairing, including Diana at AMC, from this iteration. Ben would have remained at AMC, and Diana and Frank would have had to move down their list to their fourth choice.

Second Round (Version 2)

Applicant	ROL	Program status	Match result
Ben	1. AMC	Spots tentatively filled by Amy and Diana	Tentatively no match (both members of Diana's couple have to have stable matches before Ben is permanently ousted from this position)
	2. CCH	Ben ranks higher than Frank, which dissolves Diana/Frank's entire matched pair	Tentative match (but will end up taking Diana's AMC spot)

Third Round

Applicant	ROL	Program status	Match result
Diana/Frank	1. AMC/AMC	Though Diana was ranked higher than Ben, Frank was not ranked so there is no match	
	2. BAU/BAU	One open slot; though Diana is ranked #1, Frank is not ranked higher than Charlie and thus unable to take the #2 spot so there is no match	
	3. AMC/CCH	CCH has one open slot, but Ben is preferred, bumping Frank and thus dissolving the entire matched pair	No match
	4. BAU/DDH	Both have open slots	Tentative match

Note the impact of matching as a couple. Had they matched independently, Diana would have matched at AMC and Frank would have ended up at BAU, the first and second most popular schools. Instead, they ended up at the second and fourth most popular programs.

> **Insider Tip:** Mathematically, there is no way within the confines of the algorithm for a stronger applicant to improve the desirability of the weaker applicant. Prior to initiation of the algorithm, however, a program that really wants the stronger applicant and is aware that he/she is in a couples match, may adjust their ROL to rank the weaker applicant higher than they would have on his/her own merit. However, this is incredibly unlikely and not a method on which to rely.

Diana and Frank made two wise choices when compiling their list. First, their fifth rank choice involved a "No match" for Diana (more accurately, she listed program code "999999999" as her fifth choice). While we do not necessarily endorse enlisting this option so early on a ROL, it is important to include it for demonstrative purposes. Diana is a strong candidate in a less competitive field and would have a strong chance of matching in a desirable location as part of the after-match SOAP.

> **Insider Tip:** Be aware that, after failing to match as a couple, the NRMP does *not* then re-evaluate each member's ROL as an individual. Consequently, it is wise to add a few "No match" combinations at the end of your list.

Second, they compiled a list in which Frank, in a much more competitive specialty, was willing to move down his list of preferences more quickly than Diana (while maintaining a geographic relationship). With that in mind, it is easy to see how quickly a couple's ROL can be exhausted. For couples, even more than the individual applicant, it is important to have a long ROL. The fee schedule for couples matching is the usual $65 per applicant plus an additional $15 couple's registration fee. Once registered as a couple (done by updating your profile after registering first as an individual), the couple can rank 30 programs before incurring an additional fee. To be clear, this means that 30 unique programs can be ranked as part of a pair, not 30 combinations.

> **Insider Tip:** Thirty unique programs can be listed by each member of a couple for their initial registration fee, which allows for 870 permutations ($n!/(n - r)!$), where $n = 30$ (number of programs) and $r = 2$ choices for the pair. As part of a matching pair, we recommend a lengthy ROL.

We will spend more time, in Chapter 5: *The Selection Process – Yours* and Chapter 11: *After the Interview*, discussing the facets to consider when deciding what programs will best suit your needs and how these will factor into compiling a ROL. For now, we hope that you understand the matching algorithm, and are convinced of the importance of applying to and later ranking

Chapter 1

as many programs as possible in order to increase in your chances of matching. Just as important, we hope you realize that listing programs based on your preferences, rather than what you think your "chances" are of getting in, will serve your interests rather than that of the programs.

References

1. Roth, A. E. and Peranson, E. (1999) The redesign of the matching market for American physicians: some engineering aspects of economic design. *American Economic Review* **89**: 748–780.

2. Johnson, R. (1994) The stable marriage problem: Structure and algorithms, by Dan Gusfield and Robert Irving, The MIT Press, Cambridge, MA, 1989, 240 pp., $27.50. *Networks* **24** (2): 129–130.

3. NRMP: All In Policy; available from: http://www.nrmp.org/policies/all-in-policy/ [accessed September 2014].

4. NRMP (2103) *Data Release and Research Committee: Results of the 2013 NRMP Applicant Survey by Preferred Specialty and Applicant Type*. National Resident Matching Program: Washington, DC.

5. The Prize in Economic Sciences 2012; available from: http://www.nobelprize.org/nobel_prizes/economic-sciences/laureates/2012/ [accessed March 2014].

6. Gale, D. and Shapley, L. S. (1962) College admissions and the stability of marriage. *The American Mathematical Monthly* **69**: 9–15.

7. Peranson, E. and Randlett, R. R. (1995) The NRMP matching algorithm revisited: theory versus practice. National Resident Matching Program. *Academic Medicine* **70**: 477–484; discussion 485–489.

8. NRMP: Run A Match; available from: http://www.nrmp.org/wp-content/uploads/2014/05/Run-A-Match.pdf [accessed September 2014].

Chapter 1

2: Specialty Selection – Where to Begin

S pecialty choice is a complicated interplay of student and residency program preference. The realistic probability of achieving a residency spot in a desired specialty should play a large role in your decision-making process. The next chapter (Chapter 3: *The Specialties – Program Directors' Perspectives*) discusses individual subspecialties, offering information over a broad spectrum of topics ranging from typical lifestyle and salary to a Program Director's vision of the ideal candidate. However, the selection process begins with medical student choice, which is the focus of this chapter. Once your decision is made, the remainder of the book will help you maximize your chances of successfully attaining a residency spot in your chosen specialty.

Asking a first-year medical student what they want to specialize in will likely elicit a non-chalant, "I'm not sure yet." Asking a third-year medical student will likely evoke a much more panicked, "I don't know … I don't even know what I like." A large contributor to this classic third-year frenzy is the realization that the decision-making time they thought they had in their "clinical years" is almost gone. The vast majority of your pre-clinical coursework is largely predetermined, leaving little room for actual clinical experience. This fact falsely leads students to believe that specialty choice is a decision that should be put off until their final 2 years. The reality is that most institutions require students to select their fourth-year electives by the spring of their third year. In turn, your fourth-year electives are generally directed by the field to which you wish to apply. The beginning of your fourth year is most effectively used for increasing exposure to your desired specialty in order to confirm your choice and to request letters of recommendation (LoRs) before applying in September. This means that you really only have the first 6–9 months of your third year to solidify your decision. Moreover, schools often weigh Surgery and Internal Medicine more heavily during the third-year schedule (possibly as much as 3 months each). These two subjects can take up a significant portion of your deciding time, giving you little chance to explore other subspecialties before making this critical determination.

Numerous surveys have noted student anxiety regarding specialty choice revolves around lack of knowledge of their own interests and as-yet untested abilities, lack of information about the specialties themselves, and an absence of support for the formidable task [1]. As understanding your own goals and interests is the first and most important phase in this process, we have developed the acronym, **SELF** (Figure 2.1), to help walk you through specialty selection. This simplified stepwise decision-making tool was born out of extensive research into both the cognitive process of general decision making [2–10] as well as the more specific specialty choice selection.

Self-assessment

- Structured assessment tools
  - PVIP, MSPI-R
  - Personality inventory
- Personal affiliations. Do your own interests and values better align with PC or NPC

Exploration

- **Increase exposure to a specialty**
  - *Hands off*
    - Peruse specialty list on ABMS
    - Research basic information on CIM and specialty/society/board websites
    - Attend career/specialty panels and interest group meetings
  - *Hands on*
    - Extracurricular or core curricular exposure
    - Shadowing (try to increase exposure to multiple practice settings)
    - Specialty-specific mentor
- **Understand the important characteristics of a specialty**
  - *Content*
  - *Corollary*

Likelihood

- **Competitiveness of specialty in general**
  - Position availability
  - Unmatch rate
  - Qualification of successfully matching candidates. Assess figures for initial filter
    - USMLE scores
    - Alpha Omega Alpha
- **Competitiveness of individual residency programs**
  - FREIDA Online
  - Residency program webpage (look for minimum scores and current resident Profiles)
  - Medical student forums
  - Advisors

Fallback

- Reassess parallels between specialty choice and original stated values and goals. Have priorities changed?
- Too many interests?
- Need more time to make a decision or improve application?
- Want to change specialties?

Figure 2.1 SELF: **S**elf–Assessment → **E**xploration → **L**ikelihood → **F**allback. See text for definitions of abbreviations.

Insider Tip: Specialty choice is a deeply personal and complex process. To avoid getting lost along the way, remember these basic steps to finding the right specialty: **S**elf-assessment → **E**xploration → **L**ikelihood → **F**allback.

In the last three decades, there has been a huge amount of research directed at the various aspects of how a medical student chooses a specialty. There has been an upsurge of interest in the topic with the 2010 passage of the Affordable Care Act, which will expand health insurance coverage to approximately 34 million additional people in the United States [11]. While some authors disagree about the existence of a physician shortage, contending that there may in fact be a surplus of doctors but a discrepancy between the needs of the population and the distribution of physicians both in geography and specialization [12–17], few would argue against the predicted shortage of physicians, particularly primary-care (PC) physicians, in the wake of this dramatically expanded insured population. A 2008 publication by the Association of American Medical Colleges (AAMC) projected a shortage of 46 000 PC physicians by 2025 [18]. This concern about a dearth of generalists has led to the recent resurgence of specialty choice research, with the underlying hope that better understanding of the decision-making process may be useful in guiding students to a PC role that they may not have otherwise chosen. Thus, a significant portion of the research is broken down into choosing between PC specialties, usually defined as including Internal Medicine, Family Medicine, and Pediatrics, and all other specialties considered as non-primary care (NPC). A brief appraisal of this literature will help you address the first major branching point in your decision-making process, PC versus non-PC.

The majority of the research on specialty selection examines the decision-making process from either an external or internal focus. Studies that concentrate on external motivators assess factors such as institutional culture (private versus public ownership; urban versus rural location) or factors that could be manipulated during medical education, such as the degree and timing of exposure to a specialty during medical school [19, 20]. Studies have shown that public ownership of an institution greatly increases the proportion of students entering PC [20–22]. It is unclear if this association is due to medical school applicants recognizing differences among the missions of various medical schools, with those already interested in a PC career gravitating towards programs treating underserved populations. Alternatively, for the same reasons that publically funded hospitals may attract high-quality PC faculty, they in turn influence the medical students they teach. Studies also have demonstrated a correlation between curriculum and specialty choice. In comparing the selection of Family Medicine residencies of the 1981–1989 graduates of the State University of New York, only one-fourth of whom participated in a required PC clerkship [23], twice as many graduating students who participated in the PC clerkship chose a Family Medicine residency compared with those who did not (21 versus 11%).

While these external factors no doubt play an important role in the decision-making process, research into this area alone greatly underestimates the highly contextualized process of specialty choice. We discuss these studies to call attention to any undue influence that external factors may have on an important decision made at a time when you may be feeling somewhat overwhelmed. It would be a mistake to choose a specialty based on a sense of familiarity because your particular institution offers an early 6-week clinical exposure rather than a delayed 4-week one. It is important to consider your fit with a variety of specialties, particularly those not thrust upon you as part of a core curriculum.

Chapter 2

> **Insider Tip:** Be aware of the influence of institutional curriculum and culture on your decision-making process. The environment at your home hospital may be very different from where you end up practicing.

After recognizing and accounting for the effects your institution's culture and curriculum have on your decision, it is time to consider the second category of research, which focuses on internal motivations. In other words, how does a student's *composition* influence career choice? This research forms the basis of the self-assessment, the first step in our SELF acronym, and we encourage you to seriously participate in this phase. Moving forward with specialty decision with a poorly formulated construct of your interests and priorities is often cited as the reason for switching specialties later in life. Ideally, self-assessment is performed during the first 2 years of medical school. However, if you have not already done so and are in the midst of a third-year panic, it is not too late to begin.

Self-Assessment

Most investigators have tried to categorize the nebulous "self" through structured inventories attempting to capture personality, value, and preference, while few have attempted a broader point of view. We will review both.

A multitude of personality, preference, and value assessment tools are available to guide you in deciding on a specialty, though the AAMC Careers in Medicine (CIM) website (https://www.aamc.org/cim/) is by far the most centralized data source. Medical students pursuing an MD degree gain access to the site by using the AAMC identification number obtained when using a prior AAMC service, such as the Medical College Admissions Test (MCAT) or American Medical College Application Service (AMCAS). If you no longer have a record of your ID, you can retrieve the number through the AAMC ID lookup service (https://services.aamc.org/idlookup/). Those students pursuing a DO degree are unlikely to have taken the MCAT and thus have not been issued an AAMC ID. If that is the case, seek out your schools' CIM liaison, identifiable through the website, for login information. Alternatively, as of late 2013, an individual student can purchase a subscription to the CIM website.

A great starting place on the CIM website is the Physician Values In Practice (PVIP) Scale, a 60-question, 15-minute tool that prioritizes six values – autonomy, management, prestige, service, lifestyle, and scholarly pursuits – according to a five-point Likert scale (strongly agree through strongly disagree). Remember that this is a *value* assessment tool only, not a tool for deciding on a specialty. While the value scale results posit a tendency for students choosing the same profession to prioritize values in a similar manner, it does not ensure personal satisfaction with that career choice. In addition, these same values can be found in many different specialties.

Also on the CIM website is the Medical Specialty Preference Inventory, revised edition (MSPI-R), which is a 30-minute, 150-question inventory that measures your interests on a seven-point scale ranging from low to high with regard to different aspects of medical practice (such as your desire to work with patients with incurable disease or work in a setting where treatment is decided by a team of consultants). Depending on how you rate these aspects, they will assess your probability of entering one of 16 medical specialties: Anesthesiology, Dermatology, Diagnostic Radiology, Emergency Medicine, Family Medicine, Internal Medicine, Neurology, Obstetrics and Gynecology, Otolaryngology, Orthopedic Surgery, Pathology, Pediatrics, Physical Medicine and Rehabilitation, Psychiatry, Surgery, and Urology. At this early stage, it is important to keep in mind that these are major categories in specialty selection. Included within each one are areas of subspecialization, which may be very different from the overall category, such as Hospice Care subspecialization after Anesthesiology training. There are 24 American specialty boards, which rapidly expand to 150 different disciplines when all general and subspecialty certificates are considered. Although the validity of these preference assessment tools has been documented [24–26], it can be easy to sway the results if you take the test with preconceived notions of likely specialty choices. With only limited knowledge of a specialty, it is simple to see how an inventory question relates to that specialty, so that a test-taker may consciously or unconsciously answer the questions to fit a potential specialty rather than their own true preferences. When the inventory results corroborate the specialty they were considering, it can add false confidence to a choice not yet adequately researched.

> **Insider Tip:** When answering questions on interest or value scales, try to reflect your own beliefs and priorities, not those you associate with a desired specialty. You may be surprised by the results.

Personality tests are another structured assessment tool endorsed by the CIM website. The most popular are the Myers–Briggs Type Indicator (MBTI) and the Keirsey Temperament Sorter (KTS-II), which are inter-related and dichotomously classify personality based on four dimensions: extroversion versus introversion, sensing versus intuition, thinking versus feeling, and judging versus perceiving [27, 28]. While studies show there is some modest statistical relationship between specialty choice and personality assessment tools – with students going into Family Medicine tending toward sensing, feeling, and judging type personalities – researchers speculate that the results actually "imply a skewing of the odds rather than a determination of the future" [27]. The KTS-II costs $15, while the MBTI requires a trained psychologist to administer the test. There are a wide variety of other personality tests, but none has been found to be a reliable predictor of specialty choice, likely due to their narrow focus and exclusion of motivational factors.

In an effort to truly understand the multifactorial specialty decision, several investigators have strayed from more structured assessment tools and attempted to approach the subject from a comprehensive, and at times cognitive, point of view [10, 29, 30]. With a broader approach comes broader results; however, there is notable overlap in the study findings that can help you correlate your personality and preferences to your eventual specialty choice.

One study found that PC students seemed more focused on the interpersonal contact with both patients and faculty [29]. They also were attracted to the care of the whole patient, as well as increased breadth and diversity of the clinical experience. Given this prioritization of personal interaction, it is not surprising that PC students were more likely to be influenced by role models and by their sense that PC faculty had personalities, lifestyles, and career goals similar to their own. NPC students took a more objective look at the specialty, focusing on content, particularly technical, intellectual, or problem-based. They sought specialties that valued procedures, efficiency, urgent medical care, and interventions with immediately identifiable results. NPC cited little influence by role models. Other studies demonstrated PC students were more interested in diverse patients and health problems and less interested in prestige, high technology, or procedures [30]. PC students also prefer to treat relatively healthy patients, while NPC students have a stronger propensity toward hospital-based medicine and surgery, as well as greater concerns regarding malpractice, status, and income [31].

Specialty choice has even been related to Machiavellianism [32], via psychological tests measuring inclination for personal and moral detachment in order to maximize objectivity and desired outcome in encounters with others [33]. Students who scored higher on Machiavellianism scales had poor tolerance for ambiguity and tended towards authoritarianism, reliance on high-tech medicine, and an external locus of control (the idea that events in one's life are outside their control). Those who had high Machiavellianism scores tended towards specialties with limited patient interaction, such as Radiology, Anesthesia, Surgery, or Pathology, while those who were lowest in the trait chose Internal or Family Medicine. In this sense, a high Machiavellian score can be viewed as negative or positive depending on your value system. If success in the face of the uncertainty of personal patient interactions is more rewarding to you than the more defined world of lab work, procedures, and technology, you are certainly more likely to excel in PC. However, the emotional detachment and ability to externalize culpability associated with a high Machiavellianism score may be a protective, if not essential, characteristic in those specialties that deal with critically ill patients, procedures with potentially dire outcomes, or the grave diagnoses that are an everyday occurrence for the radiologist or pathologist.

> **Insider Tip:** The first task of self-assessment begins with an honest appraisal of your personality, interests, and talents, as well as life and career goals.

Now is the time to take a candid look at yourself. Which "type" of person or patient spoke to you? Which type of practice did not speak to you? This is the time to try on different versions of yourself. Once you feel like you have a solid understanding of who you are and who you want to be, it is time to focus on the content of the specialties.

Exploration

Although you now understand the basic division between PC and NPC, you may know little about the individual specialties. If you are at this stage of exploration, begin by taking a brief look at the American Board of Medical Specialties (ABMS; www.abms.org) list of general and subspecialty certification. You may be surprised at some of the subspecialty certificates available within certain specialties, as well as the various ways to achieve the same subspecialty certificate. For instance, subspecialization in Sports Medicine can be achieved through one of six different residency tracks (Emergency Medicine, Family Medicine, Internal Medicine, Orthopedic Surgery, Pediatrics, and Physical Medicine and Rehabilitation).

When considering a specialty, be careful to avoid mental shortcuts known as heuristics. When confronted with a complex task, people often employ a representative heuristic to process options quickly, comparing a situation to a perceived prototype. Facing such a daunting list, it is tempting to rapidly eliminate potential career choices the same way. A student may think, "All we did was round and talk during my Internal Medicine rotation. I prefer to do procedures, so Internal Medicine is not for me," whereas some Internal Medicine subspecialties, such as Gastroenterology, include the performance of a significant portion of diagnostic and therapeutic procedures. This simplistic manner of thinking will lead you to eliminate specialty options due to ill-conceived and incomplete representations of that field.

> **Insider Tip:** In the early stages of specialty selection, keep an open mind and research multiple potential specialties. As you move into the clinical years, do not dismiss a core curriculum specialty before trying it. The faculty and residents will pick up your lack of interest and do little to show you the full breadth of the specialty. At the very least, you deprive yourself of an enrichment opportunity. At the worst, you do not have the opportunity to dispel inaccurate preconceived notions of what a specialty entails and how it may be unexpectedly compatible with your goals and talents.

When beginning to research a potential specialty, you can start by searching the CIM website for such basic information as a very brief description of the field, length of training, and patient profile. Data on average work week and salary may be provided, but these represent only the median of reported values and may not be typical of many members of the specialty. Overall, this information is too brief to be used to eliminate an option that you would otherwise be considering. The real value in this site section is the "additional resources" tab, which lists the societies, boards, organizations, and publications associated with a specialty. Once you have identified specialties in which you are already interested or need more information, take some time to review the society webpage. There is often a section titled "medical student," "education," or "training" that usually offers a more detailed description of the specialty and what a future trainee or practitioner could expect. Attend student specialty interest group meetings, specialty panels, or even societal conferences, which often have reduced rates or even

Chapter 2

free admittance for medical students. If you are further along in your decision making, engaging in research in your potential specialty can not only expose you to the academic side of the field, but also be an important addition to your curriculum vitae (CV). Even if this research ends up being outside your eventual specialty choice, there is often a way to relate it to your application as part of a cohesive picture of your activities (e.g., a project about education in any field can be used to solidify your claim of being a future academic). Once you have narrowed your specialty choices to a handful of strong contenders, we suggest you become Student Members of these societies. This will round out your CV and keep you abreast of the latest issues within the field, which is excellent fodder for an interview. Moreover, it is a useful way to find a mentor/advisor if your institution is lacking a suitable match.

The next step is to progress to a more active approach to specialty exploration in order to either confirm or reject your initial thoughts that this may be the specialty for you. Even during your largely academic pre-clinical years, seek out specialty-specific mentors or other faculty/ fellows/residents to shadow. During your clinical years, residents can point you in the direction of faculty who have served as excellent mentors, but during your pre-clinical years, you may need an introduction from a more senior student to those residents or clinical faculty. If this is not an option, email your advisor or a Program Director, express your interest in the specialty, and ask if he/she could help arrange a shadowing experience. Since it is likely that this would occur during the daytime, you may not be able to accomplish this until a vacation. An ideal time to pursue this option may be during your "last summer" between first and second year or during spring break, which generally do not coincide with a holiday. If one of the specialties you are considering is heavily hospital-based and in-house call is probably part of your career plan, be sure to also get exposure to this aspect of the specialty. Some suggest shadowing an on-call resident, but this may be a time when the resident is feeling overworked, tired, and stressed. Being shadowed, especially by an inquisitive observer, may add to a resident's stress level and result in your having a less-than-hoped-for experience that negatively influences your choice. Before deciding to shadow an on-call resident, make sure that he or she is pleased to have the opportunity to provide insight into the specialty. Depending on the situation, be prepared to adopt a fly-on-the wall approach and save your questions for an opportune time. You should take the same approach when shadowing attendings on more hectic schedules. Observation during daytime clinic hours allows for a much freer exchange of questions and answers, but you want to observe all potential practice settings, not just the easier ones. Regardless of the setting, remember that all of your interactions with faculty and trainees can work either for or against you when it comes to application time. Always be on the lookout for potential research options or future writers of LoRs, but above all be polite, pleasant, and positive throughout the experience.

As you increase your exposure to a potential specialty, you need to consider the *content* and *corollaries* of a field. With regard to content, evaluate the most typical day in the specialty. What exactly are you doing with your time? The corollaries of specialty choice concern the consequences of practicing in a given field, outside the day-to-day operations of your job. This encompasses a wide variety of factors and is commonly referred to as "lifestyle." However, lifestyle means different things to various people. PC-bound students who say lifestyle played a large role in their specialty choice defined it as job availability in a predetermined geographic area and a broad range of work types. Conversely, NPC-bound students felt a desirable lifestyle included control over daily work commitments and time to pursue other interests, both personal and academic [29].

As a medical student, you can never be completely exposed to the full scope of a specialty. Therefore, it is important to ask about and research your different practice options, patient mix, and pathology. For instance, an interventional radiologist can be part of a busy hospital-based group and required to be on call every third to every seventh night, but this affords the opportunity to be exposed to the latest technological advancements and exciting cases. Alternatively, you can practice in a phlebotomy, venous disease, or vascular access clinic, where you will perform shorter procedures requiring less skill, but balance that with a controllable lifestyle and little (if any) call. In Internal Medicine, a huge specialty with numerous options for subspecialization and practice, students used to avoid the uncontrollable hours of the hospital Internist. However, with the growth of the "hospitalist" as a specialty, hospital-based Internal Medicine can be practiced on a per shift basis, greatly increasing the manageability of hours and workload. In addition to asking about practice options, be aware of the difference between watching and doing. Can you actually imagine yourself dealing with the mental and physical stresses of urgent procedures in the middle of the night? Take note of the hours kept by the attending. Remember that, unlike trainees, attendings have no work hour regulations.

> ✔ **Insider Tip:** Consider both the content and corollaries of a field. The content of a field relates to the daily activities of a given specialist, while the corollaries are a broader category dominated by lifestyle issues.

Chapter 2

When assessing the *content* of a field, consider the following characteristics:
- Direct patient care versus playing a consultative role for other physicians (e.g., Radiology, Pathology)
- Degree and type of patient interaction
  - Longitudinal versus short-term care
  - Urgent versus non-urgent care
  - Involvement in the psychosocial aspects of patient care
- Patient profile
  - Age, sex (e.g., Pediatrics, Adult Internist, Geriatrics, Gynecologist)
  - Healthy (maintenance issues) versus seriously or chronically ill
- Procedures
  - Number, type, and average length
- Role of technological advancement
- Intellectual challenge

- Practice setting options
  - Urban versus rural
  - Clinic versus hospital-based
- Possibility of ancillary roles
  - Research, teaching, administrative
- Possibility for future subspecialization

When assessing the *corollaries* of a specialty consider the following:
- Remuneration
  - Geographic differences both in salary and cost of living
  - Salary variations also occur with
    - Practice setting (academic versus private)
    - Years of experience
    - Level of status achieved in your institution (e.g., partner in private practice, professorship in academia)
  - Personal indebtedness
- Reasonable work hours
  - Number of hours per week; weeks per year
  - Timing of work
    - Daytime clinic hours
    - Shift work
    - Call schedule
      - Frequency
      - Is it home or hospital-based? How likely are you to be called in?
  - Flexibility of work hours leading to autonomy in your own schedule
- Congruence with (plans for) family
- Physical intensity of the work
  - Will you spend personal time merely recuperating from your last shift?
  - Do you expect to be able to maintain that level of intensity until retirement?
    - If not, what future options do you have?
- Prestige

Some regard these topics as taboo, believing that even factoring these considerations into your specialty decision undermines your initial decision to become a doctor. However, the reality is that specialty choice is part of a life plan. While it may be difficult to conceive this notion while consumed by the tedium of medical school and living off a government loan (you do have to pay those back by the way) or the good graces of family members, personal and professional lives are neither static nor mutually exclusive.

Studies [34, 35] have demonstrated that control over work hours, or a "controllable life-style," is becoming an increasingly important factor in choosing a specialty. These investigators reviewed the specialty choices of the upper 15% of students graduating from three different medical schools over 10 years. They postulated that the upper echelons of graduates were likely to have their pick of specialties, so that any identifiable change in the distribution of specialty choice would reflect a trend due to lifestyle considerations rather than the fairly fixed content of the specialty. After dividing specialties into those that featured a controllable lifestyle (CL) – Anesthesiology, Dermatology, Emergency Medicine, Neurology, Ophthalmology, Otolaryngology, Pathology, Psychiatry, and Radiology – and those that were considered non-CL (Surgery, Medicine, Family Practice, Pediatrics, and Obstetrics and Gynecology), they demonstrated a significant increase in the percentage of students entering controllable lifestyle specialties.

Another element to consider is personal debt. Historically, studies on the influence of medical student debt have not consistently found it to be a heavily weighted factor [36, 38]. However, more recent research [39, 40] has shown that rising medical student debt and the income gap between PC and specialty care has significantly deterred students from choosing PC, where starting salaries and compensation are lower than for specialists [40].

A 2005 study reported a disinclination to enter PC when student debt exceeded $150 000 at graduation [41], yet the AAMC reported that the median indebtedness of the 2013 graduating class was $175 000, with 40% of graduates owing more than $200 000 and nearly 20% being more than $250 000 in debt [42]. As startling as these figures are, they do not reflect the total amounts of repaid loan debt, which can be two to three times higher when adding interest related to an extended repayment plan (25–30 years). For instance, a resident who opts for forbearance during a 3-year residency and then pays back that loan with standard repayment over 10 years will pay $2700 per month and accrue $151 000 in interest, for a total payment of $326 000. However, with the trend in healthcare towards specialization, the reality is postgraduate training will likely last 7 years. In this case, with a 7-year forbearance and then standard repayment, the loan will cost $3300 per month and accrue $227 000 in interest, for a total repayment of $402 000. If your physician salary does not allow for a monthly payment of $3300 and you opt for the extended 25-year repayment plan, a $175 000 loan will end up costing $1600 per month for a total repayment of $492 000. Of additional concern is the current economic climate, which has forced many lenders to drop student loans from their portfolio. Those still in the business of lending to students or residents may soon find debt burdens exceed their willingness to extend further credit, including home mortgages [43].

As grim a picture these numbers paint, before you decide that you cannot afford to pursue a career in PC, consider the following. In 2013, a model was developed for analyzing the financial viability of a career in PC under the current level of medical student debt in the context of a physician's expected household income and expenses. It examined the discretionary income of a fictional indebted physician, "Dr. Median," under various combinations of career tracks (PC physician and two higher-paying specialists: Surgery and Obstetrics and Gynecology), degree of education debt, and participation in federal loan forgiveness/repayment programs, such as the National Health Service Corps (NHSC), while accounting for either high or moderate cost of living cities (Boston versus Denver, respectively). According to this model, with median levels of debt (described as $150 000), forbearance during residency, and an aggressive 10-year repayment plan, a PC physician living in Boston with a starting salary of $145 000 would have $1100 of discretionary income per month, which increased to $1500 per month in Denver. These numbers, while not applicable to the unique situation of every PC physician, indicate that with a median level of debt, a career in PC is financially viable even when residing in a high-cost city. However, graduates with higher levels of debt likely will need to invoke additional strategies, such as extended repayment, federal loan forgiveness/repayment programs, or living in lower-cost areas. The model calculated that PC physicians under the same scenario, but with $200 000 in debt, would have only $200 per month discretionary income if living in Boston.

Another point to consider is that we are in a time of great health reform, in which reimbursement schemes may change dramatically. In the past, the concept of prestige in the healthcare field was tied to insurance carriers' reimbursement rate and, in turn, salary [10]. As reimbursement rates are typically higher for hospital-based procedures rather than clinic-based preventative medicine, a certain air of status became associated with procedure-oriented specialties. However, in 2012, the Medicare Payment Advisory Commission (MedPAC) proposed to cut Medicare reimbursement for specialists by 5.9% a year for 3 years (total of 16.7%), followed by a 7-year freeze at the reduced levels [44]. PC providers would not have their reimbursement rates cut, but would have them frozen for 10 years. Moreover, in its 2013 Report to Congress, MedPAC advised that Medicare reimbursement be immediately made site-neutral, meaning that payment for procedures performed in a hospital setting be cut to equal those performed in an outpatient clinic [45]. While these are just proposals at the time of writing this book, MedPAC's recommendations are usually harbingers of future health policy.

In the end, "times they are a-changing," so making any specialty decision based solely on salary expectations would be a mistake.

> **Insider Tip:** Insurance reimbursement and, in turn, physician income are in flux, so that salary expectations may be far from reality by the time training is complete. While income should factor into choosing a specialty, it should not be the sole deciding point.

Likelihood

After narrowing down your considerations to a few fields, it is time to consider the other side of choosing a specialty – can you get in? To get a better grasp on your likelihood of attaining a residency spot, you need to understand the competitiveness of the field. You can get this information from reviewing the most recent National Residency Matching Program (NRMP®) Results and Match Data and focusing on these specific data points:

- Number of available residency spots per applicant
- Number of applicants that failed to match in the specialty
- Mean number of programs applied to in this specialty
  Comparing this with the mean number of programs applied to in other specialties will give you the perception of the previous class regarding the competitiveness of the field compared with others

- Applicants' choice by specialty

  Did applicants get spots in their first choice specialty?

Beyond position availability, you need to develop an understanding of selection factors. The raw data for this analysis can be found in the NRMP's *Charting Outcomes in the Match: Characteristics of Applicants Who Matched to Their Preferred Specialty*. Table 2.1 is a compilation of the 2013 NRMP *Results and Data* (published annually) [46] and 2011 *Charting Outcomes* [47]. Although the latter report is not published on an annual basis, the most recent one will be more than adequate to identify some of the assets of applicants who successfully matched in their first choice specialty. We will discuss ways to underscore all of your positive attributes – quantitative and qualitative – in later chapters. However, most programs make an initial screen of the residency applications based on a few quantitative measures, most often United States Medical Licensing Examination® (USMLE®) Step 1 (if your scores are borderline, see

Table 2.1 Specialty data.

| Specialty | Specialty position availability | | | | Matched applicant characteristics | | |
	Total positions offered	Positions per US Senior	Positions per total applicants	Unmatched US Seniors (%)[a]	USMLE Step[b] 1	2	Alpha Omega Alpha (%)
Anesthesiology	1653	1.4	0.9	2.3	226	235	8.9
Dermatology	407	0.9	0.7	6.9	244	253	50.8
Diagnostic Radiology	1143	1.4	0.9	1.0	240	245	26.4
Emergency Medicine	1744	1.1	0.8	6.5	223	234	9.1
Family Medicine	3037	2.2	0.7	3.4	213	225	6.5
General Surgery	1185	1.1	0.6	10.5	227	238	13.1
Internal Medicine	6612	2.0	0.7	2.5	226	237	15.5
Internal Medicine/ Pediatrics	366	1.1	0.9	3.9	230	242	24.2
Neurological Surgery	204	0.9	0.7	16.1	239	241	25.3
Neurology	692	1.9	0.8	0.7	225	233	11.9
Obstetrics and Gynecology	1259	1.2	0.7	7.9	220	233	10.8
Orthopedic Surgery	693	0.8	0.7	18.5	240	245	27.1
Otolaryngology	292	0.8	0.7	21.5	243	250	41.6
Pathology	583	2.1	0.7	2.7	226	233	10.9
Pediatrics	2699	1.4	0.8	2.4	221	234	11.6
Physical Medicine and Rehabilitation	397	1.8	0.7	10.5	214	224	3.9
Plastic Surgery	127	0.7	0.7	11.5	249	249	45.9
Psychiatry	1362	1.9	0.7	3.2	214	225	4.6
Radiation Oncology	183	1.1	0.9	6.3	240	244	31.2

[a]US Seniors who ranked each specialty as their only choice.
[b]Around 20% of US allopathic medical school seniors do not take USMLE Step 2 prior to the Match.
Source: Data adapted with permission from [46, 47].

Chapter 2

Insider Tips throughout later chapters on how to make it beyond this step). More in-depth analysis of your application may be done after this initial screen, either before or after your interview depending on the competitiveness of the program. Other objective considerations include the number of research experiences, presentations, abstracts, and publications; a prior PhD or other graduate degree; and being a graduate of one of the 40 US medical schools with the highest National Institutes of Health funding ($100 million or more). This last measure is included because some Program Directors give preference to applicants who graduated from a research-intensive medical school. Of course, there are a number of unmeasurable components to your application, such as LoRs and personal statement, which will play a significant role in receiving an interview and/or securing a residency spot, but these will be discussed in more depth in subsequent chapters.

If you feel that you meet or nearly meet the qualifications of the standard specialty applicant, your next step is to begin assessing the competitiveness of individual residency programs. If you are slightly below the average USMLE score for your chosen residency, you can still gain access to a relatively competitive field if you are willing to be flexible regarding where you go for residency. The American Medical Association (AMA)'s online database, FREIDA Online® (Fellowship and Residency Electronic Interactive Database), can be found under the Education > Graduate Medical Education tab (http://www.ama-assn.org/ama) and includes 9500 accredited Graduate Medical Education (GME) programs that you can search by specialty, state, or training institution. In order to gain access you will need to create an AMA account. The account is free and does not require a paid membership. FREIDA Online contains basic information, such as program ID number, participation in the Electronic Residency Application Services (ERAS®) or NRMP, and how many training positions are offered. To get a sense of the competitiveness of individual programs, consult their websites. Some openly state their minimum USMLE scores; many publish CVs or profiles of their current residents. Review these to see if you have similar academic accomplishments and interests.

> **Insider Tip:** You can get a sense of how competitive a residency program is by reviewing their website. Even if they do not post their minimum acceptable USMLE score, a review of the profiles of current residents will give you an idea of the level of accomplishment of those residents who successfully matched there.

Other resources include student forums and specialty-specific websites. Of course, you should also consult your advisor, who may have knowledge of what has been required in the past to successfully match in the specialty of your choice.

Fallback

During the fallback phase of specialty selection, you should pause and take a moment to reconsider. In the complexity of specialty decision making, did you get lost along the way?

Do your final specialty consideration(s) align themselves with the values, life, and professional goals you defined in the first step of SELF or have your priorities evolved?

It is easy to get caught up in the glamour of a specialty when you first experience it. Perhaps you were attracted by the excitement of saving someone's life or by becoming immersed in a great learning environment created by an enthusiastic attending mixed with a supportive team. Before jumping into a specialty based on a single experience, be sure it will still work with your original aspirations. Or maybe your priorities have changed? Multiple studies have found that medical students have specialty change rates of 25% between matriculation and graduation, which increases to 38% when subspecialization swaps are included [48–50]. A majority of these changes are due to a shift in prioritization of financial and lifestyle considerations.

Perhaps despite a solid academic performance, you find yourself enamored with a specialty but concerned that you will not successfully match there.

The way to handle this issue depends on how different your application is from that of the average candidate. If you feel like your academic performance has been excellent but your board scores are not up to par, discuss this with a trusted advisor, who may be able to help you find solid residency programs, some which may be in less desirable locations. To get past the initial "numbers screen," you may need to direct your efforts at specific (realistic) programs. Consider audition electives and/or research with a faculty member at your desired program. Have a mentor or LoR writer make a phone call for you, particularly if they have a connection with the program (alumnus, friend, or mutual acquaintance). The remainder of this book will help you maximize the other aspects of your application and interview to ensure success once you get past this point.

If, however, your scores are way below the expectations of the specialty, phone calls, letters, and audition electives may at most grant you a courtesy interview, but with little real intention to offer you a residency position. In this case, all you have done is waste crucial time and effort. Instead, you need to consider viable alternatives. Before dismissing the idea of switching specialties – because it smells vaguely of failure, something that does not sit well with most medical students – consider that there likely are many specialties in which you would flourish. Why cheat yourself of that opportunity? Also, remember that continuing to pursue an unattainable residency will result in the more public failure of not matching. Also, a student who enters the Match and is not successful in finding a spot has a greatly decreased chance of matching the next year. Not matching is considered a "black mark," and some programs will not even consider your application or the extenuating circumstances, believing those who reviewed your application last year must have already found something egregiously wrong.

Just because you fall short of the expectations of a competitive field, you are not doomed. You still have options. First, is there is another, less-competitive residency route to the same subspecialty? As mentioned earlier, there are six different specialties with sports medicine as a subspecialty option and some are easier to match. Multiple other subspecialties have various training options. Revisit the ABMS webpage to explore your options.

Second, is there another (less-competitive) specialty in which you could be happy? You can apply to both specialties, ranking all the residency options for your preferred specialty first and then your "safer" specialty choice second. Anderson *et al.* tackled this issue in a study surveying Surgical Program Directors perceptions of the Match [51]. She found that 44% of Program Directors found nothing wrong with applying to multiple specialties and, in fact, 32.5% felt it was an unavoidable result of the Match system itself, whereas 12.1% felt it was ethically wrong, citing it "indicated a lack of commitment to surgery." Interestingly, among those Program Directors who felt there were credible reasons for applying to more than one specialty, such as "undecided on field of interest (58.7%), couples match issues (53.4%), applicant wants to ensure match (39.3%), geographic constraints (32.0%), and academically weak (27.2%)," 75.4% of Program Directors still felt dual specialty applicants were negatively ranked for doing so. If employing this approach you will need to be aware of the potentially negative consequences and work closely with your student affairs office to help mitigate them. For example, applying to two different residency programs in the same hospital may suggest to a Program Director that you are not really interested in that field and it may be better to reserve one application per institution.

Third, consider whether you could reasonably improve your application with more time, perhaps by delaying graduation or doing a preliminary year of residency in another field. You can read more about this option in the scenario below.

Maybe you have researched and experienced multiple specialties and find yourself in the enviable position of too many interests, unencumbered by academic or lifestyle considerations?

Medical students are generally of above average intelligence and may excel in and even enjoy multiple specialties. Try to articulate what you like about the specialties, which despite appearing different on the surface, may have many important similarities. Highlight the areas of overlap and turn your attention to the specialty that has the most of the attributes you emphasized in your self-assessment. If that still does not help make a decision, revisit the content and corollaries described previously. Will the fringe benefits of one specialty better suit your preferred lifestyle? Will the less competitive specialty open up more opportunities to get the residency and eventual practice location that you want? In the end, there may simply be multiple specialties in which you would be equally happy.

Perhaps you feel that you need more time because you are not yet ready or equipped to make a decision, or maybe you are starting to doubt your place in the medical field altogether.

If you are coming across this book later in your medical school training and really have not yet actively explored the specialties, we encourage you to talk to your advisor or Dean. They may offer you some options for a crash course in exposing you to a specialty, such as reworking your clinical schedule, delaying graduation, or entering a dual-degree program. However, delayed graduation is not an option universally granted by medical schools and it may incur more tuition.

Alternatively, you could pursue postgraduate medical-related employment, research, or a degree, usually an MPH or MBA. However, postgraduate employment options without completing a residency are limited. They may not cover your student loan debts, and dual degree application deadlines may have already passed. While doing postgraduate research or clinical work will not cost you another year of tuition, they have a few negative consequences.

Graduates do not fare as well in the Match as current students. For those who attended a US medical school, the NRMP reports a graduate match rate in the 40th percentile compared with the 90th percentile for senior students. In addition, you need to secure funding for research or be paid at the relatively low rate for a research assistant. This is an important factor, as many student loans enter the repayment phase upon or 6 months after graduation.

Lastly, you can do a Preliminary Year in Medicine, Surgery, or a Transitional program (a program with a mixed curriculum, often with rotations in both Medicine and Surgery). This increased clinical exposure may help you define your interests and improve your application. Successfully working as an intern alongside various attending physicians should allow you to get more meaningful recommendations from clinical staff and demonstrate your commitment to medicine. Carefully consider what type of program you enter. A robust program may satisfy the prerequisite for specialties entered as a second postgraduate year (PGY-2), such as Radiology and Psychiatry, or count as a PGY-1 year for Internal Medicine or Surgical categorical programs. That way you will not have lost any training time, while some programs do not accept a Transitional Year program as a replacement for a categorical PGY-1.

Maybe you are questioning your specialty choice and wondering if it is too late to change your mind.

It is absolutely permissible to change your mind. However, the process becomes increasingly burdensome as you advance in your training, so be sure you are swapping specialties for the right reasons. Students who switch specialties often do not describe having undergone an epiphany, but rather a shift in priorities or a correction of false initial perceptions of a field [29]. Be certain that your modified perceptions of a field are grounded in greater knowledge of its content and corollaries, rather than purely on any negative experience you may have had with classmates, residents, or faculty while on a rotation. While interactions with colleagues and patients constitute a large part of your daily work experience, recognize the environment and mood at the site where you rotated may not be representative of the entire specialty. If you feel that a negative interaction may be at the core of your desire to switch, try to arrange for rotations in that specialty at other sites before completely abandoning the specialty.

If you wish to switch specialties shortly before application time, talk to your advisor about how this will affect your chances. If you are academically strong, it may be a matter of quickly building relationships with faculty in order to get a good LoR. If you are forthcoming and courteous with your original letter writers about your reasons for switching, they may offer to put in a good word for you with your new letter writer. If you are not as strong a candidate, you may need to delay graduating or applying to the Match.

Although clearly not ideal, some people switch specialties during or after completing one residency. Although this may feel like lost time, remember that any training will be useful in your personal and professional development. Another consideration is residency funding. A hospital receives GME funds based on the length of your initial residency training. If you change your specialty and your total residency training will surpass the time/funding allotted by GME, the program or Institution will be responsible for the additional time of your training. As a consequence, some programs do not consider applicants trying to transfer between specialties. In the end, you must weigh the considerations of "lost" time against continuing on in a career in which you are unhappy.

Summary

Specialty choice is a complex task which should begin with a realistic appraisal of your own value system. This will assist you in the first branching point in the decision tree, PC versus NPC. Despite research and concerted efforts to increase the number of students entering PC fields, there are opposing trends toward further specialization, partly driven by student perceptions of greater career and lifestyle satisfaction through specialty practice [43]. However, the reality of practice and the associated lifestyle often deviate from that perception, and this may be increased during a time of great health care reform. As a medical student, you must actively participate in selecting a specialty by exploring multiple fields in the context of this changing environment, and examining the content and corollaries of each specialty. Always remember that specialty choice is part of a complete life plan.

References

1. Savickas, M. L., *et al.* (1986) Difficulties experienced by medical students in choosing a specialty. *Journal of Medical Education* **61** (6): 467–469.
2. Simon, H. (1977) *The New Science of Management Decision*, 2nd edn. Englewood Cliffs, NJ: Prentice Hall.
3. Camerer, C. F. (1991) Judgment and decision making, J. Frank Yates. Englewood Cliffs, New Jersey, Prentice-Hall Inc. 1990. *Journal of Behavioral Decision Making* **4** (1): 76–78.
4. Brichacek, V. (1973) [Mathematical psychology 1972]. *Activitas Nervosa Superior (Praha)* **15** (4): 278–286.
5. Townsend, J. T. (2008) Mathematical psychology: prospects for the 21 century: a Guest Editorial. *Journal of Mathematical Psychology* **52** (5): 269–280.
6. Keen, P. G. W. (1978) *Decision Support Systems: An Organizational Perspective*. Reading, MA: Addison-Wesley.
7. Cohen, M. J. and Olsen, J. P. (1972) A garbage can model of organizational choice. *Administrative Sciences Quarterly* **17** (1): 1–25.
8. Klein, G. (2008) Naturalistic decision making. *Human Factors: The Journal of the Human Factors and Ergonomics Society* **50** (3): 456–460.
9. Tversky, A. (1972) Elimination by aspects: a theory of choice. *Psychological Review* **79** (4): 281.
10. Reed, V., Jernstedt, G. C., and Reber, E. S. (2001) Understanding and improving medical student specialty choice: a synthesis of the literature using decision theory as a referent. *Teaching & Learning in Medicine* **13** (2): 117–129.
11. Foster, R. S. (2011) Estimated financial effects of the "Patient Protection and Affordable Care Act," as amended; available from http://www.hhs.gov/asl/testify/2011/03/t20110330e.html [accessed September 2014].
12. Schroeder, S. A. (1993) Training an appropriate mix of physicians to meet the nation's needs. *Academic Medicine* **68** (2): 118–122.
13. Schroeder, S. A. (1993) The U.S. physician supply: generalism in retreat. *Bulletin of the New York Academy of Medicine* **70** (3): 103–117.
14. Schroeder, S. A. and Sandy, L. G. (1993) Specialty distribution of U.S. physicians – the invisible driver of health care costs. *New England Journal of Medicine* **328** (13): 961–963.
15. Lohr, K. N., Vanselow, N. A., and Detmer, D. E. (eds.) (1996) *The Nation's Physician Workforce: Options for Balancing Supply and Requirements*. Washington, DC: The National Academies Press.

16. Green, L. A., *et al.* (2004) *The Physician Workforce of the United States: A Family Medicine Perspective.* Washington, DC: TRG Center.

17. The Council on Graduate Medical Education. Twentieth Report: Advancing Primary Care; available from: http://www.hrsa.gov/advisorycommittees/bhpradvisory/cogme/reports/twentiethreport.pdf [accessed September 2014].

18. Dill, M. J. and Salsberg, E. S. (2008) *The Complexities of Physician Supply and Demand: Projections Through 2025.* Washington, DC: Association of American Medical Colleges.

19. Meurer, L. N. (1995) Influence of medical school curriculum on primary care specialty choice: analysis and synthesis of the literature. *Academic Medicine* **70** (5): 388–397.

20. Campos-Outcalt, D., *et al.* (1995) The effects of medical school curricula, faculty role models, and biomedical research support on choice of generalist physician careers: a review and quality assessment of the literature. *Academic Medicine* **70** (7): 611–619.

21. Martini, C. J., *et al.* (1994) Medical school and student characteristics that influence choosing a generalist career. *JAMA* **272** (9): 661–668.

22. Whitcomb, M. E., *et al.* (1992) Comparing the characteristics of schools that produce high percentages and low percentages of primary care physicians. *Academic Medicine* **67** (9): 587–591.

23. Erney, S. L., Allen, D. L., and Siska, K. F. (1991) Effect of a year-long primary care clerkship on graduates' selection of family practice residencies. *Academic Medicine* **66** (4): 234–236.

24. Zimny, G. H. (1980) Predictive validity of the Medical Specialty Preference Inventory. *Medical Education* **14** (6): 414–418.

25. Savickas, M. B., Brisbin, L. A., and Pethtel, L. L. (1988) Predictive validity of two medical specialty preference inventories. *Measurement and Evaluation in Counseling and Development* **21**: 106–112.

26. Richard, G. (2011) *Medical Specialty Preference Inventory, Revised Edition (MSPI-R), Technical Manual.* Washington DC: Association of American Colleges.

27. Friedman, C. P. and Slatt, L. M. (1988) New results relating the Myers–Briggs Type Indicator and medical specialty choice. *Journal of Medical Education* **63** (4): 325–327.

28. Keirsey, D. and Bates, M. (1978) *Please Understand Me II: Temperament, Character, Intelligence.* Del Mar, CA: Prometheus Nemesis.

29. Burack, J. H., *et al.* (1997) A study of medical students' specialty-choice pathways: trying on possible selves. *Academic Medicine* **72** (6): 534–541.

30. Bland, C. J., Meurer, L. N., and Maldonado, G. (1995) Determinants of primary care specialty choice: a non-statistical meta-analysis of the literature. *Academic Medicine* **70** (7): 620–641.

31. Gorenflo, D. W., Ruffin, M. T. T., and Sheets, K. J. (1994) A multivariate model for specialty preference by medical students. *Journal of Family Practice* **39** (6): 570–576.

32. Merrill, J. M., *et al.* (1993) Machiavellianism in medical students. *American Journal of Medical Science* **305** (5): 285–288.

33. Christie, R. G., *et al.* (1970) *Studies in Machiavellianism.* New York, NY: Academic Press.

34. Schwartz, R. W., *et al.* (1990) The controllable lifestyle factor and students' attitudes about specialty selection. *Academic Medicine* **65** (3): 207–210.

35. Schwartz, R. W., *et al.* (1989) Controllable lifestyle: a new factor in career choice by medical students. *Academic Medicine* **64** (10): 606–609.

36. Kassebaum, D. G., Szenas, P. L., and Caldwell, K. (1993) Educational debt, specialty choices, and practice intentions of underrepresented-minority medical school graduates. *Academic Medicine* **68** (6): 506–511.

37. Fox, M. (1993) Medical student indebtedness and choice of specialization. *Inquiry* **30** (1): 84–94.

38. Spar, I. L., Pryor, K. C., and Simon, W. (1993) Effect of debt level on the residency preferences of graduating medical students. *Academic Medicine* **68** (7): 570–572.

39. Specialty and Geographic Distribution of the Physician Workforce: What Influences Medical Student & Resident Choices?; available form: http://www.graham-center.org/online/etc/medialib/graham/documents/publications/mongraphs-books/2009/rgcmo-specialty-geographic.Par.0001.File.tmp/Specialty-geography-compressed.pdf [accessed September 2014].

40. AMA (2008) *Report 3 (I-08): Barriers to Primary Care as a Medical Career Choice.* Chicago, IL: American Medical Association.

Chapter 2

41. Rosenblatt, R. A. and Andrilla, C. H. (2005) The impact of U.S. medical students' debt on their choice of primary care careers: an analysis of data from the 2002 medical school graduation questionnaire. *Academic Medicine* **80** (9): 815–819.

42. AAMC (2013) *Medical Student Education: Debt, Costs, and Loan Repayment Fact Card*. Washington, DC: American Association of Medical Colleges

43. Greysen, S. R., Chen, C., and Mullan, F. (2011) A history of medical student debt: observations and implications for the future of medical education. *Academic Medicine* **86** (7): 840–845.

44. Medicare Payment Advisory Commission (2012) *Report to the Congress: Medicare Repayment*. Washington, DC: Medicare Payment Advisory Commission.

45. Medicare Payment Advisory Commission (2013) *Report to the Congress: Medicare Repayment*. Washington, DC: Medicare Payment Advisory Commission.

46. NRMP (2011) *Charting Outcomes in the Match, 2011*. Washington, DC: National Resident Matching Program.

47. NRMP (2013) *Results and Data: 2013 Main Residency Match®*. National Resident Matching Program: Washington, DC.

48. Tardiff, K., *et al.* (1986) Selection and change of specialties by medical school graduates. *Journal of Medical Education* **61** (10): 790–796.

49. Jarecky, R. K., *et al.* (1991) Stability of medical specialty selection at the University of Kentucky. *Academic Medicine* **66** (12): 756–761.

50. David, A. K. and Blosser, A. (1990) Long-term outcomes of primary care residency choice by graduating medical students in one medical school. *Journal of Family Practice* **31** (4): 411–416.

51. Anderson, K. D. and Jacobs, D. M. (2000) General surgery program directors' perceptions of the match. *Current Surgery* **57** (5): 460–465.

Chapter 2

3: The Specialties – Program Directors' Perspectives

With the fundamental issues of career and residency choice in mind, we break down each specialty through the eyes of a residency Program Director. We include the information you always wanted to know but were afraid to ask, such as salary and lifestyle both as a resident and an attending. For each individual specialty, we give information regarding the residency application process, including competitiveness and **Insider Tips**.

While each specialty is uniquely written and presented by a specific Program Director, we have generally divided each specialty into the following subsections:

- **Introduction.** A brief overview of the specialty.
- **Preparation.** Leading up to the application process, we offer advice on what you can do to strengthen your application. For instance, what should you be doing in the pre-clinical and clinical years? Should you do an away elective?
- **Applying.** Takes a more in-depth look at the competiveness of the field, including important statistics to consider when preparing a rank order list (ROL). Also, at a certain point in your application process, there are things you cannot change about your application, such as a less than desirable board score. This section discusses the relative importance of individual objective assessments (such as board scores) and subjective measurements. Once invited for an interview, you have achieved the minimum quantitative performance scores that the program has deemed acceptable. The interview is time for the qualitative review, where the focus is on what non-numerical aspects set you apart from the other applicants. Why does this Program Director want to work alongside you for the next few years? What can you bring to the program?
- **Quick Facts.** Highlights key information of the application process from sources including the National Resident Matching Program (NRMP®) and the 2012 American Medical Group Association *Medical Group Compensation and Financial Survey*, such as match rate, degree of competitiveness (less competitive, competitive, and highly competitive), and average number of programs applied to.
- **Insider Tips.** Offers valuable insight into the residency application, as well as other important information, such as specialty-specific awards and grants that are available to medical students.

Anesthesiology

Qi Cui Ott, MD

Beth Israel Deaconess Medical Center, Harvard Medical School, Boston, MA

Introduction

Anesthesiology embodies the practices of perioperative medicine, critical care, pain management, and resource management in crisis situations. Pre-operatively, we assess patients' co-morbidities and stratify their risk for perioperative complications, optimize them for surgery, and recommend necessary modifications to the planned surgical procedure. In the Operating Room, in addition to providing optimum operating conditions for surgeons, we orchestrate the safe passage of the patient through his/her surgery by vigilantly monitoring vital signs, anticipating potential complications, and rapidly responding to adverse intra-operative events. We manage team dynamics to allow surgeons, anesthesiologists, nurses and technicians to work optimally together to provide the best care. Postoperatively, we provide critical care and pain management in the Recovery Room and Intensive Care Unit (ICU).

Anesthesiologists must have a thorough understanding of pharmacology, and a mastery of human physiology and its reactions to perioperative insults. The skill of applying this knowledge to rapidly diagnose clinical events is a common asset of all anesthesiologists. The ability to be constantly vigilant is a must, and a love for fast-paced, hands-on medicine is essential for a good fit and smooth transition into the field of anesthesiology. The field is also most suitable for physicians who are pragmatic, goal-oriented problem solvers, and those who can keep calm and think critically in times of extreme pressure and stress.

Anesthesiology is a field that supports a variety of clinical practice models and levels of compensation. If you choose to practice exclusively in the subspecialized fields of Critical Care or Pain Management, you can pursue a career completely outside of the Operating Room. In an academic practice, you may pursue other projects in conjunction with your clinical Operating Room work, such as teaching of residents and fellows, clinical or basic science research, quality improvement projects, global medicine, public health, biomedical engineering, and operations management. Clinically, you will typically supervise two residents or up to three Certified Registered Nurse Anesthetists (CRNAs) in a 40- to 50-hour work week. However, in private practice, you may supervise up to six CRNAs or work solo in MD-only practices. Your reimbursement typically is directly related to the number of hours you work and the acuity of the cases you do, although each practice has its own incentive system. Compensation, benefits, and hours vary vastly depending on the group and geographic location, but overall the salary may be three or more times that of an academic position.

Residency is 4 years long, consisting of an internship year plus 3 years of Clinical Anesthesiology. Accepted internships include most Preliminary internships in Medicine, Surgery, Pediatrics, Obstetrics and Gynecology, and most Transitional internships. Progressively more Anesthesiology residencies offer a categorical internship that meets the Accreditation Council for Graduate Medical Education (ACGME) requirements for broad education in medical disciplines. ACGME-accredited fellowships are available in Cardiothoracic Anesthesia, Pediatric Anesthesia, Obstetric Anesthesia, Critical Care, and Pain Medicine, and there are non-accredited fellowships in Regional, Vascular, and Neuro Anesthesia. All fellowships are 1 year long. Many graduates pursue a subspecialty fellowship to develop a niche or be more competitive in the job market.

Anesthesiology residencies generally ramp up resident call responsibilities according to their level of training. In most programs, the first 1–2 months is a "tutorial" period during which residents do not take overnight call, and focus on gaining competence in airway management and providing the basic anesthetic. Call structure varies greatly among residencies and hospitals. While some small hospitals have anesthesiologists who take pager call from home, most large academic centers with residency programs have an in-house attending anesthesiologist and one or more anesthesia residents. Responsibilities include perioperative management of patients undergoing urgent or emergent surgery, emergent airway management throughout the hospital's inpatient services, obstetric anesthesia on the labor and delivery ward, critical care in the ICUs, and urgent pain management consults. Once the tutorial period is over, a junior resident typically will be assigned lower acuity cases on call (such as appendectomies and orthopedic surgeries in healthy young patients) and assist senior residents on bigger cases (major vascular, emergent neurosurgery, traumas). Call scheduling also varies greatly among residency programs, depending largely on the size of the residency program and Operating Room volume. In-house main Operating Room calls may be 24 hours. Obstetrics calls may be similar or done in 10- or 12-hour shifts. Pain service calls may be taken in-house or from home.

> **Insider Tip:** When comparing residency program call duties, take into consideration not only the weight of the call burden, but also the breadth and acuity of cases to which those calls will expose you, as this greatly affects the rigor and quality of your training.

Non-call work days also vary greatly among training programs and depend on the Operating Room schedule. Typically, Operating Rooms run from 7:30 or 8 a.m. to 4:30 or 5 p.m. and a resident is assigned to a specific room each day. A typical day begins about an hour before the Operating Room start time, when the resident arrives to set up the Operating Room and prepare the patient before surgery. Electively scheduled cases typically end by 5 p.m., but if they run late, the call team may relieve the non-call resident if they are available. After relief from the Operating Room, residents have the responsibility to preview their cases for the next day and see patients pre-operatively if they are in-house. They then devise anesthetic plans for their assigned cases and discuss them with their attendings. Since residents in Anesthesiology must master a body of knowledge that is not part of the required curriculum in medical school, they can expect to spend 1–2 hours per day studying.

Chapter 3

> **Insider Tip:** Consider the balance of clinical service and educational opportunities in each residency program. Deficiencies in either can weaken the quality of your training.

While Anesthesiology residents typically work fewer hours per week than their Medicine and Surgery counterparts, many discover that the energy required to be constantly vigilant throughout the day makes them feel as though they have worked a longer day. Anesthesiology is a specialty that is suitable for those who thrive in fast-paced, high-risk, high-acuity, and skills-based environments.

Preparation

Excellent performance in the core clinical rotations (Medicine, Surgery, Pediatrics, Obstetrics and Gynecology, and Neurology) is extremely important. This demonstrates academic vigor and proof of a solid fund of knowledge upon which to base a career in Anesthesiology. A thorough understanding of, and a clear commitment to, the specialty is also crucial. An elective in anesthesia, beyond the basic requirement, is critical. Additional anesthesia electives, either in the subspecialties or at an outside institution, can be very helpful.

> **Insider Tip:** Find a way to set yourself apart on paper, knowing that most applicants to anesthesiology have an excellent academic record. Make it personal to provide substance for an interesting interview down the line. But be sincere – tall tales can backfire.

While applicants with solely a strong academic record will be reviewed, they lack the competitive edge of a well-rounded candidate who can demonstrate possession of the life skills necessary to excel in residency. Skills essential to the making of a strong Anesthesiology resident include those in leadership, team work, problem solving, adaptation in stressful situations, and social interactions and service. These skills may be demonstrated through a variety of extracurricular (and non-anesthesia) pursuits such as competitive sports, international missions, community service, college or postgraduate jobs, and hobbies. If you have cultivated certain skills that you think will make you a better anesthesiologist, we want to know. If you have not, go out and do it.

As you go through clinical rotations and extracurricular pursuits, think about cultivating professional relationships that can generate strong letters of recommendation. At least one of your letters should be from an anesthesiologist who can directly attest to your performance in the specialty. Letter writers from other specialties or from research experience should be able to comment specifically on those strengths and attributes that would make you a strong resident and anesthesiologist.

✓ **Insider Tip:** A glowing, specific, and personal letter from a lesser-known staff member is more useful than a lukewarm or generic letter from a department chair.

If you already know your top choices of residency programs, seek out opportunities to collaborate on projects with faculty who have connections to those programs or who work directly with faculty at them. Alternatively, consider an "audition elective" – doing an anesthesia elective at your preferred program. This is both a strong demonstration to the Program Director of your interest in his/her program and an opportunity for you to find an internal letter writer. Most programs look favorably on students from other medical schools who rotate through their department, and many may grant you an interview just for rotating through. Keep in mind, though, that like an audition, your performance during this elective can help or hurt you. Be prepared by reading about your assigned cases. Get there early and stay late, and be eager to work. If you are working with residents, make yourself helpful to them. Be a team player. Interact well with housestaff, faculty, and Operating Room personnel. Show them why you would be fantastic to have in the program. A strong letter from someone within your preferred program will go a long way.

Applying

In 2013, 1653 anesthesiology positions were offered at the PGY-1 and PGY-2 levels; 69.3% of these positions were filled by US Seniors and 96.2% of the total positions offered were filled. International Medical Graduates (IMGs) filled 9.8% of PGY-1 anesthesiology positions and 12.6% of PGY-2 positions. According to data from the 2012 National Resident Matching Program (NRMP®) *Program Director Survey*, the average program receives 719 applications, interviews 117 candidates, and ranks 98 candidates for a class of eight residents [1–5].

While our institution does not have a strict cutoff number for United States Medical Licensing Examination® (USMLE®) Step 1 scores, we do consider a score of 220 as the minimum to be competitive. In 2011, the mean USMLE Step 1 and 2 scores of matched US Seniors were 226 and 235, respectively. Applications with lower scores will be reviewed and consideration may be given to applicants who have made significant achievements in other areas. In these instances, we still highly encourage applicants to demonstrate an improvement in USMLE

QUICK FACTS

Rank: Competitive
Median salary: $377 375
Residency years: 4 years (including Preliminary)
Number of residency positions: 1653 (1073 PGY-1 and 580 PGY-2)
Number of filled residency positions: 1591 (96.2%)
Number filled by US Seniors: 1146 (69.3%)
Number of applicants for PGY-1:
 US Seniors: 1208
 Total: 1893
Median number of applications:
 US Seniors: 30
 Independent: 50
Median number of interviews offered:
 US Seniors: 15
 Independent: 8
Median number of programs ranked:
 US Seniors: 11
 Independent: 7
Average resident work hours: 60–70 hours
Average attending work hours: 40–50 hours
Resident call: In-house
Data based upon [1–3].

Chapter 3

Step 2 score before the interview season. Candidates successfully matching at a highly competitive residency program often have USMLE Step 1 scores of 250 or higher.

Insider Tip: Take USMLE Step 2 before the interview season if your Step 1 score is low.

According to the 2012 NRMP *Program Director Survey*, the most important factors for ranking applicants were the interactions during the interview, interpersonal skills and professionalism, class rank, and USMLE score.

Insider Tip: Every aspect of the interview day, as well as your interactions with the institution before and after the interview, is extremely important.

Once you are invited for an interview, your academic record most likely has been deemed strong enough to succeed at the program. The impression you leave at the interview is likely the most important factor in determining whether you will match at a program. The anesthesia attending and resident pair form the core anesthesia care team. Together, they face many challenging and stressful situations day and night. The staff wants to know that you will be honest and trustworthy, communicate effectively, be eager to learn and follow instructions, and are fun to work with. If at interview you display characteristics that make others unenthusiastic to have you on their team, you can be sure you will not be ranked highly.

Extra Insider Tips:
- **If a program is important to you, do not miss the dinner the night before.** Your attendance demonstrates your interest in the program and your absence will be interpreted as the opposite. Consider the dinner an interview with the residents. It is your opportunity to get a sense of "fit." You are interviewing the resident culture at that program to see if it is an environment in which you would thrive. This is a key time to gauge resident happiness and to ask questions without staff presence. Be on your good behavior – the residents are interviewing you as well. While residents will not talk to staff about your questions (they know from when they were in your shoes that this is your chance to get candid answers), they can report unprofessional behavior or alarming interactions.
- **Do your homework.** Research the residency program before you go for interview. Knowing the basics allows you to ask more in-depth questions about the program, and you will get more out of the interview for the time and money you spend going. At the same time, it serves as strong indicator to your interviewer that you are interested in the program and that you are a smart consumer.
- **Be aware of body language.** If you have not been on many professional interviews or are particularly uncomfortable in social situations, consider practicing the body

language component of the interview with close friends and get feedback. Remember that attending anesthesiologists are looking at you as a potential team member in managing life or death situations in the middle of the night. They want to know that you are someone with whom it is easy to interact and communicate.

- **Ask questions.** Be prepared to ask at least one or two questions in each interview, if given the chance. Even if you have asked a specific question already, another person may have a different perspective or provide more information. Having no questions may be interpreted as lack of interest.
- **Be professional and courteous throughout the application process.** This should go without saying. You are seeking to train as a professional – demonstrate your ability to behave professionally!

References

1. NRMP (2013) *Results and Data: 2013 Main Residency Match®*. Washington, DC: National Resident Matching Program.
2. NRMP (2013) *Data Release and Research Committee: Results of the 2013 NRMP Applicant Survey by Preferred Specialty and Applicant Type*. Washington, DC: National Resident Matching Program.
3. AMGA (2012) *Medical Group Compensation and Financial Survey*. Alexandria, VA: American Medical Group Association.
4. NRMP (2012) *Data Release and Research Committee: Results of the 2012 NRMP Program Director Survey*. Washington, DC: National Resident Matching Program.
5. NRMP (2011) *Charting Outcomes in the Match, 2011*. Washington, DC: National Resident Matching Program.

Chapter 3

Dermatology and "Med-Derm" (Internal Medicine and Dermatology)

Elena B. Hawryluk, MD, PhD, Steven T. Chen, MD, MPH, Vinod E. Nambudiri, MD, MBA, and Rachel V. Reynolds, MD
Harvard Combined Dermatology Residency Training Program, Harvard Medical School, Boston, MA

Introduction

Dermatology is one of the few fields that allows physicians to practice a medical specialty that encompasses both adult and pediatric patient care, surgery, cosmetics, and pathology, and frequently addresses a broad differential diagnosis of inflammatory, infectious, neoplastic, and autoimmune disorders. The successful dermatologist has a keen eye for visual diagnosis and pattern recognition, attention to fine points, and appreciation for rare details. The Dermatology Board Certifying Examination is among the most challenging, including slide-based pathology questions. Consequently, Dermatology residency programs are seeking applicants who have demonstrated an outstanding academic ability and aptitude through academic grades (Alpha Omega Alpha membership is common among applicants) and high board scores. The specialty is highly competitive due to rigorous academic demands, and perceived lifestyle and salary. Many programs are interested in training future academic leaders, and also value completed research and productivity.

Dermatology training is 4 years long, consisting of a Transitional Year or Preliminary Year in Medicine, Pediatrics, Obstetrics and Gynecology, Family Medicine, or Surgery, and 3 years of Dermatology residency. An additional training option is integrated training in Internal Medicine and Dermatology ("Med-Derm"), which is a 5-year dual residency, or a research track that shortens clinical training and adds dedicated research time (see below). Dermatology residency is typically comprised of outpatient clinics and inpatient consultation services. Outpatient clinical experiences span Medical Dermatology, Procedural Dermatology, and Cosmetic Training. A majority of residents enter the workforce after completion of residency, though some choose to enter fellowships (typically for 1 year) in a subspecialty such as Procedural Dermatology (Mohs Fellowship), Pediatric Dermatology, Dermatopathology, or one of the newer non-accredited programs in Lasers, Medical Dermatology, Cutaneous Oncology, Rheumatology-Dermatology, or Public Health-Dermatology.

Insider Tip: If you are considering a Dermatology subspecialty, make sure that you identify a residency program that allows early exposure to the subspecialty, as fellowship applications are required as early as the beginning of postgraduate year PGY-3 (second year of Dermatology).

Dermatology residency programs vary in the number of residents, which affects the number of call weeks per year and inpatient coverage responsibilities. Many programs start night and weekend call duties in the fall of their first year of dermatology (PGY-2), and programs differ with respect to whether the call is front-loaded in the first and second years. While largely an outpatient-based specialty, programs may include a range of inpatient consultation duties, which are sometimes conducted at the end of a full outpatient clinic day rather than having dedicated inpatient consultation time. There is often wide variation in the inpatient consult load among hospitals.

Dedicated didactic time varies among programs and one should take this into consideration when exploring opportunities for didactic versus independent learning. There is wide variation among residency programs in the autonomy of residents with surgical, laser, and cosmetic procedures. There is a broad range in the patient populations that are cared for by the program's residents and it is ideal to have clinical exposure to patients of all skin types. Another consideration is the implementation of a continuity clinic, during which a resident gains skills in ongoing patient management, often under the guidance of a single clinical mentor. Programs vary with respect to the number of elective months during residency, with a maximum of 3 months allowed by the American Board of Dermatology (ABD), and the amount of time that can be spent outside of the institution during training for exposure to other research or clinical opportunities.

Given the nature of a predominantly outpatient-based specialty, even considering the inpatient call duties, the majority of Dermatology residents work fewer hours and have more flexible time than their Medicine and Surgery counterparts. There is a substantial amount of time required to study and learn the vast literature to become proficient in the recognition of esoteric conditions. As such, much of the time spent during a Dermatology residency may not be in the clinics or hospital, but is on the resident's own time mastering the literature and preparing for the board exam at the culmination of his/her training. This flexibility makes Dermatology a specialty well-suited for residents with other commitments, whether research or personal.

There are also specialized residency types that may be appealing to applicants, such as the Med-Derm Residency or Dermatology Research Residency. There are six Med-Derm Residency Programs and eight positions were available in 2013. These programs are 5 years in duration, after which individuals are eligible for board certification in both Internal Medicine and Dermatology. The majority of programs are structured with the first year emphasizing Internal Medicine, the second year emphasizing Dermatology, and the remainder of the 3 years split equally for a total of 30 months in each field. Residents training in both Internal Medicine and Dermatology often have a special interest in the management of complex medical dermatologic conditions – ranging from connective tissue diseases to cutaneous oncology to infectious diseases – or in the management of inpatients with dermatologic disease. Graduates are able to pursue additional subspecialty training in any of the fields of Internal Medicine or Dermatology. For those considering training in Med-Derm, strong clinical exposures during medical school to both Internal Medicine and complex medical Dermatology provide

Chapter 3

important foundations, and a research interest in the area may be particularly helpful. An additional consideration one should make before applying for a Med-Derm residency is whether the combined program is necessary for his/her career goals.

A Dermatology Research Residency Program, also called a "2 + 2" or "Research Track," generally consists of an intern year followed by 2 years of full-time dermatology clinical training and then up to 2 years of research. Depending on the program and subject to ABD approval, residents in some research track programs are able to complete their formal residency training after 1 year of research and take the board exam with their matriculating class, while others take the board exam after 2 years of research. For those considering the Research Program, a strong background in research with demonstrated productivity (including publications, posters, presentations, and/or funding) is an advantage. It is a good idea to identify potential research mentors at the programs you are considering. At some programs, you must match specifically into a Research Track position, while other programs allow flexibility to declare your track after matriculation.

Preparation

Outstanding performance academically (United States Medical Licensing Examination® (USMLE®) exams) and during clinical rotations (especially Medicine, Surgery, and Dermatology) is extremely important, as is demonstrating a commitment to the specialty through research or relevant experiences. However, remember that these basic features will be common to all competitive applicants.

> **Insider Tip:** Think early about how to set yourself apart on paper. Demonstrating your interest in dermatology through projects or papers can often take a long time to complete!

Accomplishments that could appeal to a program range from significant research contributions (PhD, named research fellowship year(s), with publications, posters, abstracts, and/or talks) to substantial service experiences and significant leadership skills. There is an appreciation for productivity (in terms of papers, chapters, presentations, or other output) or contribution to one's field.

It is ideal to demonstrate one's interest in dermatology regardless of your other accomplishments, through work on a research project that is relevant to the field. Seek out faculty mentors for opportunities to spend time in the clinic, write a case report or case series, or contribute to a project. Working on a review article or case-based project is a great way to learn more about dermatology and specific diseases.

Applicants coming from medical schools with no Dermatology program should seek support from faculty who are aware of your interest in dermatology and enable you to cultivate your clinical interest during medical school. It may also be helpful to connect with a local dermatologist or neighboring institution to identify faculty mentors. The American Academy of Dermatology (AAD) lists dermatologists who are interested in serving as mentors to medical students and has opportunities available such as the Diversity Mentorship Program to foster medical student experiences working with dermatologists. Additionally, the AAD Medical Student Core Curriculum provides an excellent online platform for learning about a variety of cutaneous diagnoses.

An away elective rotation provides the opportunity to network and be exposed to another program. However, it is vital to have an outstanding rotation, as this will be considered when your application is reviewed there, and interactions with all individuals associated with the program (including residents, staff, and patients) will make an impact. For those applicants without a home Dermatology program, the away rotation is crucial not only for networking, but also for further exposure to the field. Often, these applicants will complete two to three away rotations. During an away rotation, the student is often given an opportunity to give a prepared talk during grand rounds or didactics. This is an excellent opportunity to stand out when the application season begins.

Applying

In 2013, a total of 407 Dermatology positions were offered (38 PGY-1 positions at 22 programs and 369 PGY-2 positions at 109 programs) in addition to eight Med-Derm positions at six programs. Among the 38 available PGY-1 Dermatology positions, 21 were filled by US Seniors, 13 by prior US graduates, and two by International Medical Graduates (IMGs), while one position was unfilled. Among the 369 available PGY-2 dermatology positions, 316 were filled by US Seniors, 37 by prior US graduates, and six by IMGs, with seven positions unfilled. According to data from the 2012 National Resident Matching Program (NRMP®) *Program Director Survey*, the average program receives 332 applications, interviews 33 candidates, and ranks 27 candidates for a class of three residents [1–5].

Given the highly competitive nature of applying to dermatology residency, it is important to consider all opportunities for your application to shine. USMLE Step 1 scores, clerkship grades, and academic awards provide a way to demonstrate your aptitude, so these should be taken seriously. If your application is average in these areas or otherwise lacking, it is important to distinguish yourself

QUICK FACTS

Rank: Highly competitive
Median salary: $397 370
Residency years: 4 years (including Preliminary)
Categorical and advanced positions:
 Med-Derm: 5 years
Number of residency positions: 407 (38 PGY-1 and 369 PGY-2)
Number of filled residency positions: 399 (98%)
Number filled by US Seniors: 337 (84.5%)
Number of applicants for PGY-2:
 US Seniors: 442
 Total: 574
Median number of applications:
 US Seniors: 72
 Independent: 85
Median number of interviews offered:
 US Seniors: 10
 Independent: 6
Median number of programs ranked:
 US Seniors: 9
 Independent: 6
Average resident work hours: 40–60 hours
Average attending work hours: 40 hours
Resident call: Home call
Data based upon [1–3]

Chapter 3

in other ways. In 2011, the mean USMLE Step 1 and 2 scores of matched US Seniors were 244 and 253, respectively. An average USMLE Step 1 score should be followed by an outstanding Step 2 score. At the same time, a sky-high board score alone will not be sufficient to obtain an interview at many dermatology programs.

The Electronic Residency Application Service (ERAS®) application includes listing one's work, and volunteer and research experience, in addition to publications (papers, books, posters, oral presentations). Experiences that involve leadership or provide impact on one's community are valuable and consideration is given regardless of whether the experiences are relevant to dermatology or not. It is increasingly common for applicants to spend one or more additional years during medical school doing research, which provides an opportunity to explore the field, enhance one's application through demonstration of productivity in terms of papers and presentations, and to develop a relationship with a faculty member who can write a more meaningful letter of recommendation. Many medical schools offer a 1-year research fellowship program, and national awards (such as those listed below) or other foundation awards can provide funding during a research year. Prolonged research such as a PhD does not need to be specifically related to dermatology, but applicants with this degree should be able to explain why they have chosen to pursue dermatology training and how their educational background fits into their overall training and career plans.

It is very important to have outstanding letters of recommendations. Letters written by someone who knows you well are better than those written by individuals who are well-known in the field who do not know you quite as well or a faculty member that has known you only during a 4-week rotation. Most applicants supply at least one letter from their home Dermatology program and applicants who have done 1 year or more of research should supply a letter from their mentor who is most familiar with their work.

The personal statement offers another opportunity to share a unique attribute about yourself that speaks directly to application reviewers. If you do not feel that you have a fascinating pearl to share, consider this a great chance to express your career goals. It is not necessary to tailor the statement to a specific residency program, but if there is one program to which you are particularly drawn, this is a great opportunity to share your plans. Overall, it is extremely important to ensure that your personal statement is grammatically correct without errors, as the statement should reflect a well-prepared, organized applicant.

Insider Tip: Extra proofreading for your personal statement is vital – errors in spelling or grammar reflect poor attention to detail!

If you have the opportunity to interview, congratulations! In many cases, you have demonstrated that you are well qualified for the position, so now it is important for both you and the residency program to determine if you are a good "fit." The program will take note of your ability to communicate clearly and discuss many of the attributes of your application. It is vital that you are able to discuss your application in detail; applicants who tout proficiency in a foreign language have been known to be interviewed in that language and you might find yourself sitting across the table from an expert in the subject of a case report you have written!

> **Insider Tip:** Your interactions in communicating with all individuals (residents and staff included) both prior to the interview and during interview-associated events are *very* important!

At the interview, applicants are often asked where they see themselves in their future career in Dermatology. It is important to answer honestly, as some programs are better suited to individuals who are interested in research, while others may be most appropriate for applicants interested in service-based careers. Dermatology residency interviews take a variety of formats. At some institutions, there are "speed dating" interviews where a candidate will have 12 encounters in which he/she will spend about 10 minutes with one or two faculty members. Other programs use longer interviews with key faculty lasting up to 30 minutes or panel interviews in which a candidate meets with several faculty at once to maximize the number of attendings who meet the applicants. Several institutions offer candidates the opportunity to deliver a brief presentation to an audience of faculty and applicants. If you are applying for a Dermatology Research Residency Program, be prepared for the possibility of having to present your research to core research faculty.

> **Extra Insider Tips:**
> - **Go to the dinner the night before the interview if offered, but be on your best behavior!** Your interactions with the residents are just as important as your actual interview. On interview day, many programs will check with the residents and staff about unusual interactions with applicants; it is important to be kind to all residents and staff you encounter. Skipping the dinner may cause you to miss an opportunity to get a feel for the program and have positive interactions with the residents, and may send a message that the opportunity was not important to you. If, however, you are unable to make it, programs are understanding. Just be polite when turning down the invitation and consider informing them of the reason for your absence.
> - **Be familiar with the program prior to the interview.** When asking a question, lead with a piece of information pertinent to the program (and yourself if possible), which can convey your commitment to the program and how you envision yourself contributing: "I see that Dr. Tsao has published some interesting research on melanoma, and I would be grateful for the opportunity to meet him and potentially work on this in the future." It is important to be familiar with the department Chairman, Program Director, and any notable faculty.
> - **If you go to a national meeting for networking, consider attending the AAD Annual Meeting.** Many medical students go to the AAD Annual Meeting, where there is an opportunity to present interesting cases at the "Gross and Microscopic Symposium." Look for the deadline in early September preceding the Annual

Chapter 3

Meeting. There are also smaller affiliated meetings, such as the Society for Pediatric Dermatology or Medical Dermatology Society, which offer opportunities for students to present.

- **Visit forums.studentdoctor.net or www.derminterest.org during the interview process.** The online calendar provides Dermatology interview dates and medical student forums alert applicants of the actual interview days that residency programs are offering interviews. Once you have possible interview dates, plan out a potential interview schedule, as often two schools where you want to interview may have conflicting dates.
- **Consider applying for research grants/fellowships.** Those specific to Dermatology include Medical Student Grants sponsored by the American Skin Association and the American Academy of Dermatology Diversity Mentorship Grant. Fellowships not specific to Dermatology include those sponsored by the Howard Hughes Medical Institute and Doris Duke Foundation.
- **When scheduling your interviews, consider completing all Preliminary and/or Transitional internship interviews earlier in the process.** This will allow you to save your Dermatology interviews for the latter part of the interview season, when the bulk are scheduled.
- **Be courteous to all other applicants, faculty, and staff, and never speak poorly about another program or person.** Dermatology is an extremely small field. What you say can affect you down the line at another interview, as faculty across the country talk frequently throughout the process.

References

1. NRMP (2013) *Results and Data: 2013 Main Residency Match®*. Washington, DC: National Resident Matching Program.
2. NRMP (2013) *Data Release and Research Committee: Results of the 2013 NRMP Applicant Survey by Preferred Specialty and Applicant Type*. Washington, DC: National Resident Matching Program.
3. AMGA (2012) *Medical Group Compensation and Financial Survey*. Alexandria, VA: American Medical Group Association.
4. NRMP (2012) *Data Release and Research Committee: Results of the 2012 NRMP Program Director Survey*. Washington, DC: National Resident Matching Program.
5. NRMP (2011) *Charting Outcomes in the Match, 2011*. Washington, DC: National Resident Matching Program.

Emergency Medicine

Carrie D. Tibbles, MD and Carlo L. Rosen, MD
Beth Israel Deaconess Medical Center, Harvard Medical School, Boston, MA

Introduction

Emergency Medicine (EM) became a formal medical specialty in the early 1970s. Early pioneers of the field recognized the need for a well-trained physician who specializes in the stabilization and management of all types of critically ill patients. EM physicians have the skills to rapidly diagnose and treat all types of acute emergent and urgent conditions in patients of all ages. One of the most rewarding aspects of practicing EM is the opportunity to quickly assess and intervene to stabilize a crashing patient. Emergency Departments are typically open 24 hours a day with open access to any patient, so EM physicians also have the opportunity to diagnose and treat a wide variety of medical and surgical conditions. In addition to the ability to rapidly reach a diagnosis in a patient, EM physicians perform a large variety of procedures. As Emergency Departments act as important safety nets for uninsured patients, EM physicians serve an important public health function. There are many fellowship opportunities in EM for residents who want to specialize further. The following are most of the fellowships currently offered in EM:

- Emergency Medical Services*
- Toxicology*
- Pediatrics*
- Sports Medicine*
- Critical Care
- Research
- Geriatrics

- Palliative Care
- Ultrasound
- International Emergency Medicine
- Education
- Hyperbaric Medicine
- Administration
- Disaster Medicine

Accreditation Council for Graduate Medical Education (ACGME)-accredited fellowships are denoted by an asterisk.

EM residency programs are either 3 or 4 years long. The majority of rotations are naturally in Emergency Departments; however, there are also important off-service rotations, with residents gaining experience with pregnant patients, pediatrics, surgical rotations, and in Intensive Care Units. Residencies also offer dedicated experiences in pre-hospital care, ultrasound, and toxicology. Both the 3- and 4-year programs have the same core requirements, with the main difference being the amount of elective time. While the structure of the rotations varies among programs, residencies generally provide a resident with an increasing level of responsibility for the patients in the Emergency Department.

EM offers a large number of practice options. There are hospital-based groups, private groups, and *locum tenens* options that allow for frequent travel. This flexibility permits a great variety of interesting options throughout your career. Academic careers include a wide variety of educational- and research-based roles. Resuscitation Science, Healthcare Delivery Science, Public

Health, Education, and International Health are just a small sampling of research options in EM. EM plays an important role in the response to large-scale disasters and in the pre-hospital environment working with ambulance companies. EM generally work in shifts, at all times of the day. There is the reality that you will work on some holidays and often weekends and nights in EM. There are also several positive aspects to shift work. Most EM physicians do not carry a pager when not working, allowing for greater freedom in their off time, as well as the possibility for additional academic or administrative pursuits, service work, and other outside interests. Shift work also tends to lead to greater flexibility in your long-term work schedule.

> **Insider Tip:** There is a wide variety of career paths in EM. If you are considering choosing EM, talk to lots of people. You will be amazed by the array of career options.

Preparation

Pre-Clinical Years

Excellent performance throughout medical school is important, starting in the pre-clinical years. As the practice of EM is such a broad field, every rotation in the early years has some applicability to your future practice. EM interest groups are often a great way to get early exposure to EM. One of the most important things you can do to learn if EM is right for you is to spend some time in the Emergency Department. Most EM physicians are more than happy to have a student spend time shadowing them on a shift. Some of you will have done work as an EM technician (EMT). While a great way to get some exposure to the specialty, it is certainly not expected that most students have done this. If you are considering EM, this is often a good time to get involved in a research project. It is generally preferable to do as much as possible on one solid project, rather than to start and not finish, or to be only peripherally involved in a number of projects.

> **Insider Tip:** An Emergency Department is a unique practice environment. The only way to truly assess if EM is for you is to spend some time in the Emergency Department.

Clinical Years

During your clinical years, while your EM months will be the most important, every clinical rotation matters, particularly your core clerkships in Medicine, Surgery, Pediatrics, and Obstetrics. Do not use your entire fourth year to pile on EM-based rotations. Pick your EM rotations carefully, based on where you potentially would want to do a residency, and plan on doing only two or three. Use the rest of your fourth year to gain deeper exposure in areas that will be important for your future practice, such as Ophthalmology, Dermatology, Cardiology, ENT (ear, nose, and throat), Anesthesia, and Critical Care.

✔ **Insider Tip:** If you are really interested in a specific residency program, you should rotate there if possible. If you are considering many options, you may want to consider rotating in programs that are very different from each other to have as a reference point for comparison. For example, rotate at a 3-year and a 4-year program or at one that is university-based and one that is located at a county hospital.

✔ **Insider Tip:** Your clinical grades are the most important part of your application. EM requires strong clinical and communication skills, the ability to successfully care for all types of patients, as well as to collaborate with different types of specialists. Most programs will look carefully at how you did on all your required clinical clerkships, not only your EM months.

✔ **Insider Tip:** Make sure on every rotation that you demonstrate that you are the kind of person we want on our team. Take initiative with your learning. Be reliable. Be truthful. Put the interests of your teammates above your own and put the interest of your patients above everything.

Applying

In 2013, 1744 EM positions were offered at the PGY-1 level; 81.9% of these positions were filled by US Seniors and 99.8% of the total positions offered were filled. International Medical Graduates (IMGs) filled 5.2% of PGY-1 positions. According to data from the 2012 National Resident Matching Program (NRMP®) *Program Director Survey*, the average program receives 719 applications, interviews 132 candidates, and ranks 117 candidates for a class of 11 residents [1–5].

Who Should Write My Letters?

The Council of Residency Directors in Emergency Medicine has developed a standard letter of evaluation/recommendation that is used by most Clerkship Directors, core faculty, and Program Directors in EM. This letter details both your performance on your EM clerkship as well as their assessment of your suitability for EM and their prediction of your success as an EM resident. Most Program Directors consider this letter to be the most

QUICK FACTS

Rank: Competitive
Median salary: $297 500
Residency years: 3–4 years
Number of residency positions: 1744
Number of filled residency positions: 1741 (99.8%)
Number filled by US Seniors: 1428 (81.9%)
Number of applicants:
  US Seniors: 1640
  Total: 2430
Ratio of applicants to available residency positions: 1.4:1
Median number of applications:
  US Seniors: 33
  Independent: 40
Median number of interviews offered:
  US Seniors: 17
  Independent: 8
Median number of programs ranked:
  US Seniors: 12
  Independent: 7
Average resident work hours: 60–70 hours
Average attending work hours: 40–50 hours
Resident call: In-house
Data based upon [1–3]

Chapter 3

important for your application. It will be noticed if you did not get a letter from an EM rotation. When selecting your other letter writers, chose faculty who know you well and can speak in depth about your positive characteristics. While it may seem desirable to obtain a letter from the Chairman, it is not essential in EM and may not add value to your application if the person does not really know you. After your EM letters, the rest should be from faculty who know you well and can speak to your unique characteristics, your clinical skills, and whether you would be fit for a career in EM.

> **Insider Tip:** During an EM clerkship, you will potentially work with a large number of faculty. Try to identify early a faculty member who may be a good choice to write a letter for you. Do not be shy about asking them up front about this possibility. Ideally, you should have two letters from faculty at two different institutions to show that you have done well on different EM rotations. Academic faculty, such as Program Directors or Medical Student Rotation Directors, are the best people to write letters of recommendation.

How Many Programs Should I Apply To?

It really depends on your unique situation and the competitiveness of your application. The most important thing you can do is find an advisor in EM who is both knowledgeable about the specific programs and willing to help you honestly assess your application. EM is a very popular choice among graduating students and has become increasingly competitive. That being said, if you have a solid application you do not need to over apply, particularly to programs where you do not have a sincere interest in potentially matching. Programs have limited interview spots and, as Program Directors, we would much rather use those slots for candidates who are seriously considering our program. While there are a myriad of high-quality programs in EM across the country, some are more competitive than others. If you are a strong applicant, but only apply to three of the top programs, you run the risk of not matching. Alternatively, as a strong applicant, you could spend a lot of money and time traveling to 35 programs and wasting time on ones in which you are not truly interested. Good advising by an experienced Program Director or EM Clerkship Director is the best method to ensure you do not err in either direction. In general, the average EM applicant visits 15–20 programs during the interview season. This should be a mix of your most desirable programs, perhaps some that may seem like a reach, and some safety options. If you visit a program where you truly do not want to work, do not put it on your rank list, as the match is a binding contract. The good news is that most US Seniors match in one of their top three choices.

Should I Take United States Medical Licensing Examination® (USMLE®) Step 2 Early?

Your USMLE Step 1 score is what most programs primarily consider. In 2011, the mean USMLE Step 1 and 2 scores of matched US Seniors were 223 and 234, respectively. If you did not do well on USMLE Step 1, an improved Step 2 score will be helpful. If you did well on

USMLE Step 1, you should schedule Step 2 at a time that makes sense for you. It is important to know that several states have a USMLE Step 2 requirement before they will issue you a training license, so know the rules in the states where you are applying.

Are There Important Differences Between 3- and 4-Year Programs?

Outcome studies of graduates of 3- and 4-year residency programs have not found any significant differences between them. In general, 4-year programs tend to be more geared towards training academic physicians, although there are many graduates of 4-year programs who practice community medicine, and several 3-year programs are very academic. Some students who are already looking to fellowship training will chose the 3-year residency as a base. It is more important to look at the focus and nature of the program than to differentiate based solely on the length of training. Many applicants interview at both 3- and 4-year programs, concluding in the end that this is often not the most important consideration.

Interviews

What Should You Expect During Your Interview?

While the specific format varies among programs, there are several common features. There is often a chance to meet informally with the residents, either the night before or after the interviews. Make every effort to attend these if possible. It is a great way to get to know the residents and ask lots of questions. Understand that you are on stage even during this casual get together. Program Directors will often hear of any unusual behavior by an applicant during the dinner. Relax and be yourself and get to know the residents who may become your long-time colleagues, but recognize that this is part of the interview process.

During the interview day, you will likely get an overview of the program from the program leadership. Then you will have a series of interviews with faculty and the Program Director. Some programs also have residents and nurses interview applicants.

> **Insider Tip:** Do your homework. Know the basics of the program before interviewing. It will allow for a much better conversation with the Program Director and faculty if you already know the basics and have well-formulated questions.

What Are We Looking For in an Applicant?

Do you know what our specialty is about? Do you have a realistic assessment of the specialty and good reasons for choosing it? Do you appear as a team player, with strong communication skills and a great attitude? Does your application have evidence of someone who is committed to patients and works well with nurses? Do you demonstrate a commitment to EM, teachability, and a willingness to work hard? We are looking for applicants who are accomplished and bright, but not arrogant. We recognize that most students do not have a long-term plan worked out at this early stage, but if you have some idea of where you see yourself several years in the future, you will likely have the opportunity to discuss this as well.

Insider Tip: Remember that the whole time you are visiting a residency program you are "on-camera," not just during your official interviews. On interview day, we always ask the residents to report strange or unpleasant personal interactions with applicants, at lunch or during the hospital tour.

What Should I Look For During the Interview Process and How Do I Pick a Program?

Selecting a residency program is ultimately a personal decision. In EM, there are outstanding training programs in every region of the country. Geography is typically the most important factor for most applicants. You want to train in the area of the country that is the most appealing to you. For many, that is remaining or returning to an area that is familiar and where you have family and friends. For others, residency is an ideal time to explore an entirely new place.

Most importantly through the interview process, you should carefully reflect on your own priorities and choose the program that best aligns with the things you care the most about. If you have a specific fellowship in which you are interested, choose a program that has a strong track record for putting residents in that fellowship. If international work or flight opportunities are really important to you, choose a program where this is a particular feature.

Insider Tip: EM has many interesting avenues to pursue and many EM physicians have multiple interests. If you are a student interested in several aspects of EM and unclear about your ultimate fellowship or career choice, choose a program that has a diverse faculty with opportunities for broad exposure across all the key areas of EM.

Below are some criteria and questions that may help you differentiate among programs:
- **During the interview, what do you think when you look at the residents?** Would you like to be like them some day?
- **How does the program feel to you?** Does it match your learning style? Do the residents and faculty seem like people with whom you would work well?
- **What is the role of the EM resident on the off-service rotations?** Rotations where you are a peripheral team member tend not to be as educational as rotations where you are an integral part of the team.
- **Is there clearly increasing responsibility in the Emergency Department as you progress through residency?** For example, many residencies have a unique supervisory role for the senior residents. Given that you will be managing an entire department upon graduation, it is very helpful to have this experience in your training.

- **Know what you are particularly interested in; do not assume that you can simply create opportunities to do whatever you want in residency.** If international medicine is important to you, make sure that is part of the program.

> **Insider Tip:** If you can manage it, try and spend some time shadowing in the Emergency Department in any program you are strongly considering. Most programs are very open to this, and it is one of the best ways to get a true sense of the program.

Conclusion

EM is a rewarding field that appeals to people who enjoy high-adrenaline situations, working in teams, and a large amount of variability in their practice. You need to love working with all types of patients and working closely with nurses and collaborating with all other specialties in the hospital. You must have excellent communication skills, creative problem-solving skills, and strong technical abilities. The field has grown in exciting ways over its brief history and offers residents many interesting career paths. Applying for residency in EM is an exciting opportunity to be part of this vibrant community. Paying attention to the advice of mentors, knowing your own priorities, working hard in medical school, and doing your homework regarding the practice of EM are the essentials to being a successful applicant in EM.

References

1. NRMP (2013) *Results and Data: 2013 Main Residency Match®*. Washington, DC: National Resident Matching Program.
2. NRMP (2013) *Data Release and Research Committee: Results of the 2013 NRMP Applicant Survey by Preferred Specialty and Applicant Type.* Washington, DC: National Resident Matching Program.
3. AMGA (2012) *Medical Group Compensation and Financial Survey*. Alexandria, VA: American Medical Group Association.
4. NRMP (2012) *Data Release and Research Committee: Results of the 2012 NRMP Program Director Survey*. Washington, DC: National Resident Matching Program.
5. NRMP (2011) *Charting Outcomes in the Match, 2011*. Washington, DC: National Resident Matching Program.

Chapter 3

Family Medicine

Robert P. Bonacci, MD, Jacob Erickson, DO, and Mary Lally, BMBCh
The Mayo Clinic, Rochester, MN

Introduction

Family physicians assume the responsibility for providing and coordinating the total health-care needs of patients and their families. It is a specialty often chosen for its breadth of scope, offering care to patients of all ages, and thus family physicians are highly self-motivated and life-long learners. Family physicians are at the front lines of medicine and are often the first physicians to evaluate a patient. Strong observational and people reading skills are essential. One can often make the diagnosis simply by listening closely and observing patients.

In some parts of the country, Family Medicine is thought of only as an outpatient specialty. However, there are many opportunities to work in other settings such as Inpatient Medicine, Obstetrics, Urgent Care, and Emergency Medicine. Additional training in these areas can offer "specialization" within Family Medicine. Family Medicine continues to be a popular specialty due to high job demand, ability to personalize careers, and flexibility of work-life balance, including the ability to practice in any geographical location.

Family Medicine residencies are traditionally 3 years long. However, some programs are beginning to adopt a 4-year curriculum. This recent trend is an answer to both national restrictions on resident work hours and the continuously expanding scope of practice that makes up Family Medicine. Most graduates of Family Medicine residencies go directly into practice. However, among the fellowships that are currently available to graduates are Sports Medicine, Obstetrics, Geriatrics, Urgent Care/Emergency Medicine, Palliative Care, Rural Medicine, and Research/Faculty Development. When choosing a residency, the following are questions you should ask to determine whether a specific program in Family Medicine is the right fit for you:

- ***Why* are you are going into Family Medicine?** Do you enjoy being the first to evaluate a patient? Do you feel this is where you can personally have the biggest impact in medicine? Does it fit with your desired lifestyle? Do you want a family-oriented specialty? Do you want to practice abroad? Do you like a wide variety of areas of work?
- **Ultimately, in what *type of practice* do you see yourself?** Examples include private practice, academics, rural, overseas medicine, and specializing within Family Medicine.

Reminding yourself of the answers to these questions will help when asking, "Will a program give me the specific training I desire?" This will save you a lot of time and headache when sifting through hundreds of potential options.

Looking at the situation broadly, Family Medicine residencies can be divided into two categories: academic-based versus community-based. Academic or university-based programs tend to be located in large teaching hospitals. These often have a multitude of resources available in terms of teaching, research, and specialist access. As these programs have multiple residencies, there can be competition for learning opportunities due to the number of residents under one roof. Most academic institutions are also referral centers, and therefore have a large volume of high-acuity patients and procedures. Community-based programs tend to be located in smaller hospitals (though this is not always the case). Residents in these programs are well trained and are sometimes the only residents in the entire hospital. Consequently, these programs potentially provide many opportunities to participate in various procedures and assume extra responsibilities. However, it is very important not to get trapped into only looking at academic *or* community programs, as these pros and cons are not true across the board. Therefore, focus your efforts on identifying a residency program that will help *you* to achieve *your* personal goals, regardless of whether or not it is in an academic or a community setting.

Bear in mind the location of your residency, as you will be living there for at least 3 years. Residents often settle relatively near to where they train, although this is certainly not always the case. If your dream is to practice in the middle of a big city, it may be a good idea to consider urban residencies; if you aspire to set up shop in a small rural community, then do not forget to consider this when you are choosing where you hope to train.

Another question that usually arises is "what is the obstetrical training like?" Obstetrical training opportunities vary widely across residencies, with some programs having large numbers of cases and even requiring additional months in this area. If you have specific dreams of performing cesarean sections in addition to practicing obstetrics, be sure to check whether individual residencies provide sufficient training experience, as many programs are encouraging that this be done as part of a fellowship after residency.

All Family Medicine residencies have required rotations in both inpatient and outpatient settings, but there can be a significant difference in the amount of time devoted to each. Decide what you are hoping for in practice, and then take this into consideration during your search. Consider the call structure, since some programs have adopted a modified call schedule and others utilize a night-float system. Ask about each to see which seems to fit you best. When interviewing, do not forget to observe how happy (or unhappy) the current residents are with their system.

Preparation

Having a well-rounded application is essential for being a strong candidate in Family Medicine. Solid academic performance as a medical student is important, especially in rotations in Family Medicine and in closely related areas such as Internal Medicine, Pediatrics, Obstetrics, and procedural-based roles. Showing dedication to the field of Family Medicine is crucial. This is often done through additional electives and subinternships, shadowing experiences, or research. As part of your application, be sure you meet the minimum requirements for each program. Have at least one letter of recommendation written by a Family Physician with whom you have worked.

Chapter 3

Make yourself stand out. Do something extra in medical school; be a member of a group, volunteer, change policy, create models for learning, find a cause. Also, do not stick only to medicine; keep up your hobbies and interests. Find a new one if you are running low. Family practitioners tend to be "people" people as well as academics and scholars, so do not be afraid to show this side of you.

Applying

In 2013, 3037 Family Medicine positions were offered at the PGY-1 level; 44.6% of these positions were filled by US Seniors and 95.9% of the total positions offered were filled. International Medical Graduates (IMGs) filled 35.4% of PGY-1 positions. According to data from the 2012 National Resident Matching Program (NRMP®) *Program Director Survey*, the average program receives 907 applications, interviews 72 candidates, and ranks 52 candidates for a class of six residents [1–5].

In a recent NRMP survey of Family Medicine Program Directors, 34% reported that they required a target United States Medical Licensing Examination® (USMLE®) Step 1 score for a candidate to receive an interview. In 2011, the mean USMLE Step 1 and 2 scores of matched US Seniors were 213 and 225, respectively; 42% of Program Directors indicated they would often consider candidates who failed USMLE Step 1 on their first attempt, while 54% seldom would.

> ## QUICK FACTS
>
> **Rank:** Less Competitive
> **Median salary:** $219 362
> **Residency years:** 3–4 years
> **Number of residency positions:** 3037
> **Number of filled residency positions:** 2914 (95.9%)
> **Number filled by US Seniors:** 1355 (44.6%)
> **Number of applicants:**
>   US Seniors: 1583
>   Total: 5946
> **Ratio of applicants to available residency positions:** 2:1
> **Median number of applications:**
>   US Seniors: 17
>   Independent: 50
> **Median number of interviews offered:**
>   US Seniors: 14
>   Independent: 8
> **Median number of programs ranked:**
>   US Seniors: 9
>   Independent: 6
> **Average resident work hours:** 50–60 hours
> **Average attending work hours:** 50–60 hours
> **Resident call:** Variable
> *Data based upon [1–3]*

In preparing you application, be sure to consider the following:
- Highlight honors received, such as Alpha Omega Alpha and a Gold Humanism Award.
- Have your Electronic Residency Application Service (ERAS®) application complete and ready for review within the first 1–2 weeks that residency directors have access to applications.
- Carefully follow any specific program instructions, such as having a letter from a practicing family physician if this is required.
- Remember that each program reviews applications differently and values different aspects of the application.

Extra Insider Tips:

- **Strongly consider an away rotation.** If you are strong clinically and have a great personality, but do not look so good on paper, this rotation could "make" it for you. A great away rotation can decrease the importance of board scores that are not so impressive.
- **If you get an interview, the program believes you are qualified to train there.** The interview is about showing off your personality and how well you gel with the program. This is *key*, since for most applicants the interview either seals the deal or breaks it. Do not underestimate how big of an impact the interview has on your chances of being ranked highly.
- **Be memorable.** Both during your interview and especially in your application, you must find a way to stand out (in a good way).
- **Keep in touch with the program, otherwise, they could, and will, forget about you.** This is especially important if you rotate with a program early in the year. After your interview, keep in touch periodically with program contacts. Be upfront with everyone if you really want to go to their program.

References

1. NRMP (2013) *Results and Data: 2013 Main Residency Match®*. Washington, DC: National Resident Matching Program.
2. NRMP (2013) *Data Release and Research Committee: Results of the 2013 NRMP Applicant Survey by Preferred Specialty and Applicant Type*. Washington, DC: National Resident Matching Program.
3. AMGA (2012) *Medical Group Compensation and Financial Survey*. Alexandria, VA: American Medical Group Association.
4. NRMP (2012) *Data Release and Research Committee: Results of the 2012 NRMP Program Director Survey*. Washington, DC: National Resident Matching Program.
5. NRMP (2011) *Charting Outcomes in the Match, 2011*. Washington, DC: National Resident Matching Program.

Chapter 3

General Surgery

Shushmita M. Ahmed, MD and James N. Lau, MD
Stanford University School of Medicine, Stanford, CA

Introduction

General Surgery is a specialty defined by direct intervention, a multidisciplinary team approach, leadership, and innovation. Indeed, one of the most appealing aspects of surgery is the ability to cure through anatomic manipulation. The true surgeon, however, is much more than a masterful technician. He/she must have a comfortable command of both the perioperative management and surgical technique to achieve the most successful outcomes for the surgical patient. Thoughtful use of adjuncts such as imaging, laboratory results, and other diagnostic modalities guide the best course of action. Therefore, surgeons must be comfortable and facile in reading and interpreting these results on their own. The surgeon is a member of the Operating Room team, and must constantly balance teamwork and leadership. Finally, in light of the invasiveness of the field, there is a constant push for improvement in skill, technique, and innovation. The profession requires that one be aware of and adaptable to changes to ensure the highest quality care at all times. Consequently, it is no surprise that General Surgery residency programs are very selective in choosing individuals who meet these criteria.

Contemporary general surgeons usually focus on a particular field and may require additional experience in the form of fellowships. Rural surgeons practice more endoscopy and gynecology, while those in a more urban setting may have trauma and general surgery call responsibilities in addition to their elective, usually abdominal, practice. The acute nature of some of the diseases and medical entities encountered by the surgeon requires a thorough anatomic, physiologic, and pathophysiologic understanding combined with the confidence to physically intervene when necessary. The development of the clinical decision-making ability in surgery requires experience that is gained by a longer residency and, at times, the need for a fellowship. Surgeons are usually the definitive care specialists in a medical system. They are relied upon to attempt to solve problems when no other avenues or specialists are available. All these aspects of surgery contribute to the demanding nature of the work and life of a modern general surgeon.

The need for general surgeons ensures job availability in virtually any setting. Within private practice, most general surgeons work as part of a group or, if in a solo practice, collaborate to lighten the call burden. Academic surgeons divide their time between teaching, research, and clinical duties. The average work week for an attending consists of 50–60 hours, exclusive of call demands. General Surgery is a demanding field; therefore, students must have a clear understanding of the expectations of the career before embarking on this path.

Surgical residency consists of 5 years of clinical training. Major academic centers offer or require 1–2 years of research or professional development activities. These research years are typically offered between the second and third (or third and fourth) years of training, depending on the institution. Fellowships encompass a broad range of fields including: Acute Care Surgery, Breast, Cardiac, Colorectal, Critical Care, Hepatobiliary, Minimally Invasive, Pediatric, Plastic, Surgical Oncology, Thoracic, Transplant, and Vascular Surgery. These fellowships typically range from 1 to 3 years. There are now integrated programs (combining General Surgery with a subspecialty) within the fields of Cardiothoracic, Plastics, and Vascular Surgery, thereby making these fellowships more sparse and competitive. These integrated programs take students directly into their programs to train in these subspecialties from the beginning of their residency.

The intern year is focused on teaching perioperative management of the patient and introducing the neophyte surgeon to basic operative skills. Nationally, interns log an average of 70–80 operative cases per year. During postgraduate year PGY-2, residents take more responsibility for diagnosing and working-up patients by seeing consults in the hospital and the Emergency Room. This allows them to develop their triaging, time management, and diagnostic skills. PGY-2 and PGY-3 also allow for more clinical autonomy and leadership while focusing their skills on the care of the critically ill. Most of the Emergency Room and Intensive Care Unit experiences occur during PGY-2. During the fourth and fifth clinical years, residents take on the role of leader (senior or chief resident). In this capacity, they assume major clinical and Operating Room decision-making responsibilities, and are the primary surgeons alongside the attending. According to Accreditation Council for Graduate Medical Education (ACGME) guidelines, surgical residents must complete at least 750 major cases throughout their 5 clinical years of training, with at least 150 major cases during the chief year. A new American Board of Surgery requirement is that 250 cases must be completed by the end of PGY-2.

In adherence to ACGME guidelines, interns are limited to 80 hours per week, including call. Twenty-four-hour duties and home call are allowed starting in PGY-2. Residents work an average of 6 days a week. During the work day, residents are involved in perioperative management, seeing patients in clinic, operating, and attending teaching and clinical conferences. All senior residents, when serving as the service chief, are expected to present in weekly Morbidity and Mortality conferences. Most residencies have a weekly simulation or skills session in addition to a didactic clinical knowledge program that helps prepare the residents for skills performance and medical knowledge assessments like the American Board of Surgery In-Training Exam (ASITE). In addition to the 80 hours per week in the hospital, residents are expected to read and prepare for the upcoming operations.

Despite the rigors of the residency, General Surgery offers a satisfying career for those willing to take the challenge. General Surgery is an ever-changing field, and advances in disease management and technology keep the work fresh. The diversity in job settings allows individuals to find their niche. Most importantly, the level of trust a patient must have to allow a surgeon access to their body creates a patient/physician relationship that is quite special and unique to this field.

Chapter 3

Preparation

Surgical management relies on a combination of qualities and skills. Therefore, excellence is sought in all clinical rotations, especially Medicine and Surgery. During Surgery rotations, one should take ownership of patients so that the team can rely on the student as a primary provider. Many students who desire a particular institution choose to do away rotations to showcase their stamina and skill set. The away rotation is equally important to the applicant to gauge the atmosphere and rigors of the program. This is also a way for applicants to ensure that they truly love the specialty and not merely the environment of surgery at their home institution.

Insider Tip: When visiting residency programs, be sure to talk to the residents as well as the faculty. Residency is a long road, and it is important to be at an institution where you have colleagues and mentors who inspire and support you.

General Surgery is a competitive residency. Many applicants take time off from medical school to pursue research. Publications and presentations at conferences demonstrate academic prowess. Activities displaying one's leadership and teamwork skills should be highlighted. However, an applicant is defined by more than his/her academic accomplishments. Therefore, remarks in evaluations regarding one's character and interpersonal skills are also instrumental in identifying a desirable resident.

Strong letters of recommendation are crucial to completing a successful application. Applicants should seek mentors within the surgical field (and preferably ones with whom they have completed a rotation) who can provide testimony to the student's strengths. It is important to meet with one's own institution's Surgery Program Director and/or Surgery Chairperson early to allow him/her the chance to not only know you as an applicant, but also be aware of your goals/wishes for residency. Program Directors and Surgery Chairpersons can be powerful allies. Department leaders of various institutions are familiar with each other, and a call from the applicant's home Program Director and/or Chairperson may turn the outcome in his or her favor. In addition to away rotations, national surgery conferences provide another venue for students to meet surgeons/mentors from other institutions. In particular, the American College of Surgeons (ACS) holds a special conference for medical students at their Annual Clinical Congress. During this conference, students receive application tips and have the opportunity to meet various Program Directors throughout the country to learn about the respective programs. Best of all, the conference is low cost to allow maximal accessibility. Some medical schools sponsor students interested in surgery to the clinical congress. Check with the core Surgery Clerkship Director at your institution to see if they or your surgery interest group support some students to defray the cost of the travel. Those unable to attend the conferences can go to the ACS website, where opportunities for remote mentorship are available.

Applying

According to the National Resident Matching Program (NRMP®), 1185 General Surgery categorical positions were offered in 2013. Of those, 1180 positions (99.6%) were filled; 954 (80.5%) positions were filled by US Seniors and 122 (10.3%) positions were filled by International Medical Graduates (IMGs). While new positions have been added every year, almost 100% of General Surgery categorical positions have been consistently filled over the past 5 years. According to data from the 2012 NRMP *Program Director Survey*, the average program receives 623 applications, interviews 68 candidates, and ranks 42 candidates for a class of five residents [1–5].

A 2013 study showed that the most important factors in choosing a General Surgery resident were United States Medical Licensing Examination® (USMLE®) Step 1 scores, publications, and personal statements [6]. Alpha Omega Alpha membership and USMLE Step 1 scores were the only variables predictive of being ranked in the top 5. In 2011, the mean USMLE Step 1 and 2 scores of matched US Seniors were 227 and 238, respectively. For applicants who have less than 230, it is important to take USMLE Step 2 early, as a significant rise in score can greatly improve the applicant's chance of receiving an interview. While published work holds the greatest weight in attesting to an applicant's research accomplishments, submitted works to be published, oral presentations, and poster presentations should also be mentioned. A unique personal statement is undoubtedly impressive. However, since most personal statements chronicle similar themes, it is more important to write something concise and sincere.

QUICK FACTS

Rank: Competitive
Median salary: $370 024
Residency years: 5 years (1–2 years research based on institution)
Number of residency positions: 1185
Number of filled residency positions: 1180 (99.6%)
Number filled by US Seniors: 954 (80.5%)
Number of applicants:
  US Seniors: 1295
  Total: 2415
Ratio of applicants to available residency positions: 2:1
Median number of applications:
  US Seniors: 38
  Independent: 77
Median number of interviews offered:
  US Seniors: 16
  Independent: 4
Median number of programs ranked:
  US Seniors: 12
  Independent: 5
Average resident work hours: 80 hours
Average attending work hours: 50–60 hours
Resident call: In-house
Data based upon [1–3]

Insider Tip: Anything on the application, however trivial, is fair game for interviewers to query. Therefore, make sure you are comfortable talking about everything that is included in your application. If you cannot talk about it, best to leave it out.

Extra Insider Tips:
- **Go to the dinner/reception the night before the interview if offered, but be careful!** This is a great opportunity to see the residents and/or faculty and their interactions with each other. Your interactions with the residents and/or faculty may

be just as important as your actual interview. Skipping the dinner/reception the night before is usually without negative consequences, so if you feel that you would not be at your best or are uncomfortable in social situations, consider finding a good excuse to miss it.

- **Be familiar with the program prior to the interview.** When asking a question, it should be specific to the program and its uniqueness. For example, reference the source and then ask if there is updated information about where the current chiefs are going to fellowship and whether it was their first choices.
- **Be confident without seeming egotistical.** Sometimes what you project is more important that what you say.
- **If you have done a subinternship at the program where you are now interviewing, make a point to see those with whom you worked, but interview with other important faculty if possible.**
- **Contact the programs you loved after you interview.** Email the Program Director and/or Chairperson (if you met them on your interview day) of the programs that you loved. Honestly tell them that you want to go there and (briefly) why it would be good for you and them. Also follow up with them after you completed all your interviews. It may seem pushy, but if interested in you, they want to know that you are interested in them.

References

1. NRMP (2013) *Results and Data: 2013 Main Residency Match®*. Washington, DC: National Resident Matching Program.
2. NRMP (2013) *Data Release and Research Committee: Results of the 2013 NRMP Applicant Survey by Preferred Specialty and Applicant Type*. Washington, DC: National Resident Matching Program.
3. AMGA (2012) *Medical Group Compensation and Financial Survey*. Alexandria, VA: American Medical Group Association.
4. NRMP (2012) *Data Release and Research Committee: Results of the 2012 NRMP Program Director Survey*. Washington, DC: National Resident Matching Program.
5. NRMP (2011) *Charting Outcomes in the Match, 2011*. Washington, DC: National Resident Matching Program.
6. Stain, S. C., *et al.* (2103) Characteristics of highly ranked applicants to general surgery residency programs. *JAMA Surgery* **148** (5): 413–417.

Chapter 3

Internal Medicine

Michaela Restivo, MD and David Chong, MD
Columbia University College of Physicians and Surgeons, New York, NY

Introduction

Internal Medicine doctors ("Internists") specialize in the prevention, diagnosis, and treatment of disease in adults. The internist is the classic form of the doctor – someone who specializes in thinking about the entire patient with the ability to manage acute and chronic disease of any organ system. Internists are problem solvers and diagnosticians, who spend their days integrating knowledge of anatomy, physiology, and pathophysiology with the environmental, social, and behavioral aspects of health. This culture of inquiry creates an atmosphere of intellectual curiosity that leads to discovery. Therefore, Internal Medicine doctors are often at the forefront of basic science, translational, clinical, epidemiological, and health policy research.

You will often hear that if you do not like rounding then Internal Medicine is not for you. In fact, inpatient practice is just a small part of Internal Medicine. The full breadth of knowledge and skills of an Internal Medicine doctor allows graduates to pursue a variety of careers after residency training, including careers that may not have a single minute spent rounding! The variety of potential career paths informs Internal Medicine Program Directors to look for well-rounded applicants with varied academic and artistic interests that reflect not only an advanced intellect, but also an ability to empathize with patients and understand the socioeconomic and behavioral aspects of health.

While 20–25% of internists remain generalists and focus on outpatient primary care or inpatient hospitalist medicine, approximately 60–75% of internists eventually subspecialize in one of the growing number of the following areas recognized by the American Board of Internal Medicine (ABIM):

- Adolescent Medicine
- Allergy and Immunology
- Cardiology
- Critical Care Medicine
- Endocrinology
- Gastroenterology
- Geriatric Medicine
- Rheumatology
- Hematology
- Hospice and Palliative Care Medicine
- Infectious Diseases
- Nephrology
- Oncology
- Pulmonary Disease
- Sports Medicine

The variety of subspecialty options allows for a broad range of career and practice types. Some Internists choose primarily interventional fields (e.g., Interventional Cardiology and Gastroenterology), while others spend most of their time in office-based, non-interventional fields (e.g., Primary Care, Endocrinology, and Allergy and Immunology).

Given the number of Internal Medicine doctors required by the healthcare system and the variety of clinical settings in which they practice, the competitiveness of Internal Medicine residency varies significantly by program and location.

Internal Medicine residency is 3 years long. Training consists of a combination of inpatient medicine wards, Intensive Care Units, an outpatient primary-care continuity clinic, and time spent pursuing additional clinical rotations, elective research, or quality projects. Some residency programs offer specialty research, primary-care, quality, or clinician educator tracks during residency. These tracks typically offer specialized mentoring and some dedicated time to pursue these interests during residency, though the exact requirements vary significantly by program. Many residents will go on to pursue fellowship training. The duration of this training varies by the fellowship subspecialty and the amount of time spent on research, but can last 1–5 years. Thus, the full duration of Internal Medicine training ranges from 3 to 8 years after medical school.

Insider Tip: As Internal Medicine offers such a wide variety of clinical paradigms, it provides a unique opportunity to incorporate other related interests into your career, including research, education, health policy, and quality/patient safety.

Preparation

Pre-Clinical Years

Success in Internal Medicine requires a working knowledge of a large breadth of material, so that it is crucial to make the most of your pre-clinical years. The knowledge gained during this time provides the basis for understanding the physiology, pathophysiology, and pharmacology that will drive clinical decisions throughout your career. Many schools use a pass/fail grading systems for the pre-clinical years – this means that really the only way to assess the relative knowledge acquired during this time is the United States Medical Licensing Examination® (USMLE®) Step 1 exam. Rather than a 1-month endeavor, you should begin to study for USMLE Step 1 from the first day of medical school. USMLE grades, especially Step 1 scores, are extremely important and often normalize medical school grades among schools. Although not perfect, USMLE scores predict those residents that will pass the ABIM Boards on the first attempt and all residencies strive to have a 100% pass rate. Research is not an absolute requirement to get into a competitive Internal Medicine residency program. Nevertheless, activities that reflect intellectual curiosity provide great material for discussion on the interview trail and will give you an opportunity to show off your medical knowledge and experience.

Insider Tip: Internal Medicine program administration is full of people who have been in your shoes – we know when you pursued research just to add it to your curriculum vitae (CV) or whether you did it because you were actually interested and really made an effort. Similarly, sort through your activities and consider removing those that seem irrelevant to your career and your pursuit of medicine (e.g., your membership in your high school stamp club or the one day you spent at the local soup kitchen). Interviewers and Program Directors will read every aspect of you application. Come to your interview ready to speak intelligently and passionately about your work, prior experiences, and any lessons learned. Just putting work on your application is not enough!

Insider Tip: Internal Medicine residency programs are frequently among the largest in the hospital. In order to fill a large number of spots, residency application committees are required to read many applications. This frequently requires use of basic objective measure cutoffs to quickly compare a large number of applicants. We therefore heavily consider scores on the USMLE exam scores and grades on third- and fourth-year clerkships to determine whom we invite for interviews. So make sure you study!

Clinical Years

While we are obviously most interested in your grades on medicine and your medicine subinternship, we also care about how you interact with teams in general, so every rotation is important! If you do not do well on your medicine third year clerkship, make sure to impress on your medicine subinternship. Clerkship grades integrate the input of a variety of sources – among these sources are your ward attendings and residents. Just like your Operating Room time is your opportunity to impress your surgical attendings and residents, rounds are your opportunity to show your medicine attending and resident that you are working hard and reading. Make sure you know the plan for your patients every day, and offer to look up any questions that come up on rounds and present the answers the following day. Take initiative and offer to help whenever you can. Most importantly, remember you are part of a healthcare team so your goal is to advance care for the patient, not to look better than anyone else on the team!

If you are certain you are interested in medicine, consider using your elective time to fill in gaps in your knowledge or weaknesses in your clinical skills. Take time to learn as much you can in the Ophthalmology and Dermatology clinics and spend time reviewing your basic Radiology and Pathology. In most cases, this is your last chance to really spend intensive time cultivating the skills of non-medicine topics – make the most of it! If you are unsure if Internal Medicine is for you, take some time to rotate through medicine clinics or rotate on ward services to see if the people you work with and the topics you contemplate are interesting to you.

Insider Tip: Medical school is 4 years and there are inevitably challenges that arise during this stressful time. If you had a personal challenge that affected your performance, be prepared to discuss this at your interview. Consider a discussion with your Dean or mentor as to whether this should be a part of your formal personal statement and Medical Student Performance Evaluation as well. Full disclosure is required if there is any interruption in training and highly encouraged for a good and fair ranking process.

Chapter 3

Applying

In 2013, 6277 Internal Medicine positions were offered at the PGY-1 level; 49.9% of these positions were filled by US Seniors and 99.4% of the total positions offered were filled. International Medical Graduates (IMGs) filled 41.0% of PGY-1 positions. According to data from the 2012 National Resident Matching Program (NRMP®) *Program Director Survey*, the average program receives 1908 applications, interviews 172 candidates, and ranks 106 candidates for a class of 10 residents. In 2011, the mean USMLE Step 1 and 2 scores of matched US Seniors were 226 and 237, respectively [1–5].

As you can see from the statistics above, there are certainly enough available Internal Medicine residency spots for all applicants. The key to matching in medicine is identifying an appropriate list of programs. Select a faculty member or Program Director with knowledge of Internal Medicine graduate training programs to critically review your application and give you a sense of the types of programs for which you are most competitive. Consider including a few programs that are slightly more competitive and some that are slightly less competitive than your current institution.

QUICK FACTS

Rank: Competitive
Average salary: $224 417
Residency years: 3 years
Number of residency positions: 6277
Number of filled residency positions: 6242 (99.4%)
Number filled by US Seniors: 3135 (49.9%)
Number of applicants:
   US Seniors: 3710
   Total: 11030
Ratio of applicants to available residency positions: 1.8:1
Median number of applications:
   US Seniors: 25
   Independent: 94
Median number of interviews offered:
   US Seniors: 15
   Independent: 9
Median number of programs ranked:
   US Seniors: 10
   Independent: 8
Average resident work hours: 80 hours
Average attending work hours: 50–60 hours
Resident call: In-house
Data based upon [1–3]

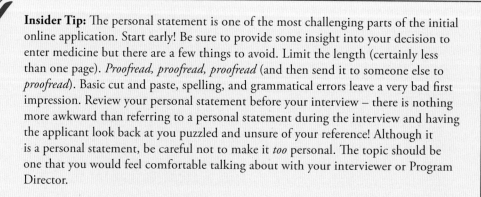

Insider Tip: The personal statement is one of the most challenging parts of the initial online application. Start early! Be sure to provide some insight into your decision to enter medicine but there are a few things to avoid. Limit the length (certainly less than one page). *Proofread, proofread, proofread* (and then send it to someone else to *proofread*). Basic cut and paste, spelling, and grammatical errors leave a very bad first impression. Review your personal statement before your interview – there is nothing more awkward than referring to a personal statement during the interview and having the applicant look back at you puzzled and unsure of your reference! Although it is a personal statement, be careful not to make it *too* personal. The topic should be one that you would feel comfortable talking about with your interviewer or Program Director.

Chapter 3

Interview Day

The exact organization and content of your interview day will vary a bit by program, but you can expect to attend a conference, spend time on ward rounds or talk to residents, receive an overview of the program, and finally have the interview. Keep in mind that you are being watched and evaluated throughout the day. Remember to show up on time! Act interested (even if you are not), do not yawn or fall asleep, hold doors open for others, and say please and thank you whenever appropriate. As you will soon learn, the world of medicine is smaller than you might expect – keep this in mind when you discuss prior interviews or programs on the interview trail with other applicants, residents, former residents, and administrative staff. Word spreads quickly, and it is not rare to hear feedback about applicants' activities and behavior on the interview trail. Your interactions with housestaff, administrative staff as well any email correspondences are all considered in the final ranking process!

Frequently Asked Questions

Qualifications/Applications

- **I did not honor in medicine, should I just stop now?** Absolutely not, keep going! Try to schedule your subinternship early in your fourth year and ace it so that you have a second evaluation of your performance for residency programs to review. It may also help to get a letter of recommendation (LoR) from your subinternship attending to reinforce your abilities and hard work.
- **Is it okay to have a faculty member outside of the Department of Medicine write me a LoR?** Absolutely. We certainly want to see one or two LoRs from Internal Medicine faculty, but if you have a mentor from a different department who knows you well, certainly also his or her letter. It is important that you choose someone who knows you well and can write you a strong letter. A short, impersonal, form letter from a very prominent faculty member is often a very big "red flag" for the recruitment committee.
- **I am applying in two specialties, is it okay to mention this?** No one likes to be someone else's second choice, so do not advertise that Medicine is not your first choice. If your application is filled with Orthopedics rotations and research, you may want to consider how best to address concerns on the interview trail about your passion for medicine.

Choosing Programs/Distinguishing Features

- **All of these programs look pretty similar, what are some of the distinguishing features?** It is true that Accreditation Council for Graduate Medical Education (ACGME) requirements for training programs have led to a similar constellation of rotations and call schedules. There are, however, some differences among programs that will affect your experience. Consider what you are looking for when it comes

Chapter 3

to the predominant patient population, program size, number of hospitals, research opportunities, autonomy and an approach to graded independence, and distribution of overnight call. Think about your career goals and review both faculty and recent graduates and fellowship lists to see if the program has successfully guided people into their desired career path.

- **What is a primary-care track? If I do a primary-care track, can I still subspecialize?** The exact nature of the primary-care tracks varies among programs. Some offer increased outpatient time for primary-care residents, while others simply offer additional mentorship opportunities. Only a very few primary-care tracks require that you commit to time as a primary-care doctor after residency; in the vast majority of categorical programs, you can still subspecialize.

- **Some programs mention having a block schedule for my clinic, what does that mean? What affect does that have on my schedule?** There are some programs that have instituted a block schedule for their outpatient continuity clinics. These schedules usually have a set number of weeks on the wards, followed by a set amount of time in the clinic (e.g., 4 weeks on the wards followed by 2 weeks in clinic – "4 + 2" schedule). There are pros and cons to this new schedule – ask around on the interview circuit to decide which you prefer.

Interview Day

- **Should I write thank you letters? Thank you emails?** You are absolutely *not* expected to send a letter through snail mail as a thank you. Some of the very competitive programs strongly discourage communication of any type after the interview, including email. For most programs sending an email is acceptable though not necessary. Do not be surprised if your email goes unreturned – the interviewers, Associate Program Directors, and Program Directors are incredibly busy and get a very high volume of thank you emails, so they are unlikely to respond to yours.

- **Should I tell my first-choice program that it is my first choice?** There is no downside to telling your first-choice program that you ranked them first. The programs cannot ask you where you ranked them. However, the community of Program Directors is small enough that they communicate among themselves, so do not tell two places that they are your first choice!

- **I know that I want to subspecialize. Should I say that on my interview?** Go for it – but remember you are applying for Internal Medicine residency, not Cardiology fellowship, and your interviewers may not be trained in your subspecialty of interest. Make sure you show enthusiasm for general Internal Medicine!

- **I do not know if I want to subspecialize. Is it okay to say that on my interview?** Absolutely! Many Internal Medicine residency applicants are undecided about fellowship and nearly all applicants change their mind during residency.

References

1. NRMP (2013) *Data Release and Research Committee: Results of the 2013 NRMP Applicant Survey by Preferred Specialty and Applicant Type.* Washington, DC: National Resident Matching Program.
2. NRMP (2013) *Results and Data: 2013 Main Residency Match®.* Washington, DC: National Resident Matching Program.
3. AMGA (2012) *Medical Group Compensation and Financial Survey.* Alexandria, VA: American Medical Group Association.
4. NRMP (2012) *Data Release and Research Committee: Results of the 2012 NRMP Program Director Survey.* Washington, DC: National Resident Matching Program.
5. NRMP (2011) *Charting Outcomes in the Match, 2011.* Washington, DC: National Resident Matching Program.

Chapter 3

Neurological Surgery

Joseph Kapurch, MD and William Krauss, MD
The Mayo Clinic, Rochester, MN

Introduction

Neurological Surgery ("Neurosurgery") is the field of medicine concerned with the prevention, diagnosis, treatment, and rehabilitation of disorders affecting the human nervous system. Neurosurgeons are trained with the expectation of becoming experts in diseases involving the brain, spinal column, peripheral nerves, and associated vasculature. The specialty encompasses a wide range of acuity, technical ability, and fast-advancing knowledge.

Neurosurgeons, by nature, are very detail-focused individuals, but they often need to make decisions which have broad implications for patients and their families. Neurosurgeons interact with many other specialties. It was once said that, sooner or later, every extremely sick hospitalized patient will get a neurosurgery consult. Like most hyperboles, it has some basis in fact.

By its very nature, Neurosurgery is a time-consuming and sometimes highly stressful vocation. All neurosurgeons are required to make difficult and ambiguous decisions, lead life-and-death discussions, and become intimately familiar with failure. Conversely, they are a unique group privileged with an ability to relieve suffering, save lives, and positively impact their communities.

Much like a surgical capacitor with a huge voltage differential, the practice of Neurosurgery includes equally massive positive and negative charges (if not so physics-inclined, you can substitute the overused roller coaster simile). To participate, you do not have to stick your fingers in sockets (or attend amusement parks); but, in the words of the immortal Ms. Frizzle, you need to be willing to take chances, make mistakes, and get messy. It is not a job for cowards or quitters.

The pop culture stereotype of a neurosurgeon is an imperious egotist who views himself as an elitist *brahmin* who condescends to help the afflicted (i.e., Alec Baldwin's character in *Malice*, albeit a cardiac surgeon). While the field's founding fathers may have lent some credibility to this, the current cadre of neurosurgeons is as varied and colorful as the instrumentation they put in patients' spines. Almost all personality types can be found in any neurosurgical training program. Additionally, multiple subspecialties have formally developed, catering both to surgeons' interests and personalities:

- Neuro-oncology
- Pediatric Neurosurgery
- Spine
- Functional/Epilepsy
- Peripheral Nerve
- Cerebrovascular/Endovascular
- Skull Base

This diversity enables surgeons to tailor their practices to help accommodate their passions, both neurosurgical and extracurricular. One can focus on high-risk vascular cases, physically demanding scoliosis corrections, simple degenerative spine, tumor resections, and any combination thereof. Procedures can take from under 30 minutes to well over 10 hours and include techniques as delicate as cerebrovascular suturing to heavy-duty spinal carpentry, sometimes in the same case. Additionally, due to their very particular set of skills, neurosurgeons have the sole ability to procure human neurologic tissue, which affords a unique asset to many basic science labs, creating valued partnerships that can be balanced with busy clinical practices. After residency, one can stay academic, developing a niche practice with relevant research opportunities, or venture into the world of private practice, serving their community and working toward one's own ambitions.

Residency

Due to the expansive and unique scope of practice, Neurosurgery was one of the earliest specialties to separate from General Surgery and develop a tailored residency program. With a minimum 7 years of training, Neurosurgery attracts and requires a special kind of student who is passionate, patient, and persevering. The first year is an infolded internship that includes up to 6 months of dedicated neurosurgical rotations with the other months incorporating Neurology, Critical Care, and vestiges of General Surgery/Trauma/Emergency. After this, the majority of the remaining 6 years is Clinical Neurosurgery, with most programs offering 1–2 years of dedicated and flexible research time. Most of a resident's job is spent in the hospital operating and managing inpatient services with a smattering of outpatient clinical rotations to round out the educational experience.

Unlike most TV portrayals, surgical residents work very hard (and they do not wear special-colored scrubs or goof around with medical colleagues for several hours a day). The new work restrictions of 80 hours per week may have made the actual term "resident" historical and obsolete, but neurosurgical trainees frequently make the most out of these temporal limitations. The exact pattern and order of different rotations varies from program to program, but all surgical training works on the principle of graduated responsibility. The postgraduate year PGY-1 initiates a gradual transition from thinking like a student to acting as a practitioner. Trainees become exposed to neurosurgical diseases and procedures, and learn the fundamental technical skills of a surgeon. As the years progress, residents spend more time learning to perform more complex neurosurgical operations and have greater autonomy in managing emergency consults. In the final years, residents assume nearly full responsibility for the neurosurgical services, with some programs even providing transitional roles in which the chiefs operate independently as junior faculty.

The training for all surgical specialties is longer than non-surgical ones, largely because the technical skills of surgery take time to develop. As with any physical act, the key to performance is practice. Neurosurgical training can be particularly arduous because it deals with some of the sickest patients, and follows the unpredictable rhythms of trauma, surgical complications, and other emergencies. However, as any senior surgeon will attest, repetition and redundancy are essential to training, and the busier one is, the better he/she will be.

Chapter 3

Insider Tip: Do not rule out a career in Neurosurgery because residency seems too hard – it is only 7 or 8 years. However, if you are worried about this, you should probably change either your mindset or career ambitions, because surgery is hard. That is part of the fun. If it were easy, everybody would be doing it.

Preparation

Pre-Clinical Years

Aside from general growth as a human being and your introduction to physicianship, the major importance of these years rests in preparation for the United States Medical Licensing Examination® (USMLE®) Step 1 examination and exposure to your Neurosurgery Department. An excellent USMLE Step 1 score is not essential to a successful match, but most Program Directors find it a useful benchmark for two reasons: (1) proof you learned something during your first 2 years of medical school, and (2) you are able to dedicate yourself to completing an unenjoyable task simply because that is what you are supposed to do. With multidisciplinary medicine and the legal advantage of specialty consultations, the first point has become less important in the actual practice of Neurosurgery. The second point, however, directly applies to surgical training. The virtues of prolonged concentration, self-sacrifice, and commitment are the *sine qua non* of a successful resident.

Without the time constraints of clinical rotations, the first 2 years of medical school are also a great time to introduce yourself to the Neurosurgery Department. The easiest way is to seek out a potential faculty mentor and pester them until they meet with you or point you toward a more receptive colleague. This initial relationship can be based on simple availability, clinical scope, or even similar athletic rooting interests and often develops into a gateway to Neurosurgery. If you are not too annoying, this then leads to shadowing in clinic, scrubbing into cases, and research opportunities with residents. This last benefit is probably the most important, since most residency programs appreciate research experience and projects often take years to develop, so getting involved early is a great advantage.

 Insider Tip: Worry not if you are late to the Neurosurgery table and do not have any publications by the time you apply. Curiosity, passion, and perseverance are the real barometers of any medical student research experience. If you were involved in projects from other departments, these should be proudly discussed and Program Directors will apply the appropriate metric to score them relative to Neurosurgery (kidding!)

Clinical Years

Unlike your Medicine colleagues, these years are actually pretty straightforward for neurosurgical applicants – do well in everything, do more well in Surgery, and do most well in the

Neurosurgery subinternships. Of course, Alpha Omega Alpha with all Honors looks good, but as anyone who has gone through the M3 year knows, those grades are sometimes more arbitrary and frustrating than an NFL overtime game being decided by a coin toss. Program Directors remember this and take grades with several pinches of salt. Truly the best attitude a medical student should have is the desire to develop a strong clinical background in all aspects of medicine. We are a privileged population, one that becomes intimately familiar with people at their weakest moments, and we should honor these varied experiences as the cornerstones of our overall physicianship.

Every time residents and faculty meet to discuss applicants, a cacophony of opinions arises about the merits of one candidate over another, this accomplishment compared to that award, blah, blah, blah. All applicants have many great qualities and the match list often becomes an Orwellian ranking of people as "more equal than others." A consensus on greatness is rarely reached, but the process of elimination is much easier. Ten out of 10 neurosurgeons agree that being a "gunner" is a strict exclusion criterion. The backstabbers are readily apparent on subinternships, but often reviews and letters from outside rotations can also give hints. As with life, the Golden Rule applies to Neurosurgery applications: do not be a jerk. You should work hard to develop a reputation as a team player, someone who makes those around him/her better. More important than a reputation, though, you should actually *be* that kind of person. Surgery is a team sport and over seven long seasons, everyone wants to have teammates that genuinely support them. The other tightrope is to talk just enough – not too much and not too little. No one likes a windbag; however, they need to know that you are alive.

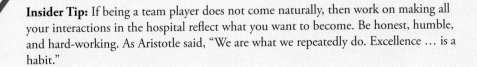

Insider Tip: If being a team player does not come naturally, then work on making all your interactions in the hospital reflect what you want to become. Be honest, humble, and hard-working. As Aristotle said, "We are what we repeatedly do. Excellence … is a habit."

Applying

In its annual statistical report, the National Resident Matching Program (NRMP®) reported that in 2013, Neurological Surgery had 99 accredited programs, offering 204 positions to start training at the PGY-1 level. There were 241 US Senior applicants and 73 independent applicants (total = 314). That works out to 1.5 applicants for every position, with 93% of US Seniors matching successfully. In 2011, the average USMLE Step 1 score for matched US Senior neurosurgery applicants was 239 and Step 2 was 241. Of successful applicants, 12% had a PhD, 28% were Alpha Omega Alpha, and more than 90% were involved in research. According to data from the 2012 NRMP *Program Director Survey*, the average program receives 188 applications, interviews 35 candidates, and ranks 24 candidates for a class of two residents [1–6].

Neurosurgery is obviously a competitive field in which to match. In fact, for what it is worth, in 2013 it was the third most competitive, behind Dermatology and Plastic Surgery. As with anything, though, scores and numbers give a solipsistic and incomplete view of the match process. In accordance with what makes most competitive people successful, many applicants get caught up on these objective markers. Typical questions include:

QUICK FACTS

Rank: Highly competitive
Median salary: $656 250
Residency years: 7 years (including PGY-1)
Number of residency positions: 204
Number of filled residency positions: 203 (99.5%)
Number filled by US Seniors: 190 (93.1%)
Number of applicants:
    US Seniors: 241
    Total: 314
Ratio of applicants to available residency positions: 1.5:1
Median number of applications:
    US Seniors: 46
    Independent: 91
Median number of interviews offered:
    US Seniors: 22
    Independent: 12
Median number of programs ranked:
    US Seniors: 15
    Independent: 8
Average resident work hours: 80 hours
Average attending work hours: 80 hours
Resident call: In-house
Data based upon [1–3]

- **My USMLE Step 1 score was 220. Should I quit?** No. Many other factors can supersede a below-average board score. However, this is an initial screener for most programs. The cutoffs vary, but many will probably be somewhere around the high teens or low twenties. Truthfully, a score below 230 will make things more difficult for an applicant, but it is not by any means a death sentence. 239 is an average, so for every score above it, there must be some below. Also the USMLE standards for foreign graduates and second-time applicants are typically higher than those for US Seniors. If you are in any of these positions, you will need to make a positive impression in some other way. You may be excluded from top-tier programs. However, some of the best neurosurgeons did not train in "top-tier" programs. Whether this be research, clinical rotations or something else, your faculty mentor can probably provide you with more concrete advice.

- **I did better on USMLE Step 2. Does that change anything?** No. Some programs require this, some consider it, but most do not even have it available by the time they interview. The major problem with USMLE Step 2 is that some applicants take it and some do not by the time decisions are made. Consequently, it is impossible for Program Directors to use it as a measuring tool.

- **How many programs should I apply to?** A good rule of thumb is 40–50, as a sliding scale based on your overall application strength (i.e., your USMLE Step 1 score). Again, your faculty mentor can help place you on this spectrum. Most importantly, do not rank a program you would not attend. Murphy's law dictates that is where you will match. And, if you do not take that position, you have violated the match agreement and become a match pariah.

Interviews

Aside from any subinternships, this is the most important part of the application process. Grades and scores can become trivial when compared to the glory of an awesome interview. Similar to not being an over-aggressive student, a big no-no in interviews is blatant bragging about yourself. Remember, most applicants have a lot of truly remarkable things on their curriculum vitae (CV) and committees can read about your awards. The two worst interviewees are either boring or cocksure. What they want to hear are the interesting side stories to your accomplishments, your passions, your ability to have a conversation, and what kind of person you are. The best approach to an interview actually is the old cliché "be yourself." The exception is if you are a complete weirdo – then keep that quiet.

Multiple forums exist for the actual interviews. Some are panels, some one-on-one, and some even with multiple applicants. The content and formality also change frequently. The most successful interviewees are the ones able to gauge an atmosphere quickly and adapt their responses. An interview with a young pediatric attending fresh out of fellowship will likely have a much different tone than one with an emeritus professor who was trained by Cushing.

> **Insider Tip:** Remember that the whole time you are visiting a place you are "on-camera," not just during your official interviews. On interview days, faculty will ask residents, nursing staff, secretaries, janitors, just about anyone to ferret out any bad interactions or things that may hint at an unseen, unpleasant side to an applicant. Dress well. Sometimes, a school tie or a school ring will win points. Avoid controversial topics, especially politics. Remember that most programs struggle with duty hour regulations, even if there is general agreement that physician fatigue is a problem. Therefore, the best attitude to have about duty hour regulations is to consider them a necessary evil.

Program Directors and faculty are definitely looking for the nascent leaders of Neurosurgery, future superstar alumni that they can boast about at meetings. However, they are also looking for people they want to work with, colleagues they will spend countless hours teaching and relying upon. Residency interviews, and the application process in total, can be very stressful. Keep in mind, though, that you are also interviewing the program. You need a program to pick you, but they also need applicants to want them. The interviews are a valuable chance to ask honest questions about a program and to see if it aligns with your priorities. Be humble and enjoy the process. It is a special experience and will go by very quickly.

References

1. NRMP (2013) *Data Release and Research Committee: Results of the 2013 NRMP Applicant Survey by Preferred Specialty and Applicant Type.* Washington, DC: National Resident Matching Program.
2. NRMP (2013) *Results and Data: 2013 Main Residency Match®.* Washington, DC: National Resident Matching Program.

Chapter 3

3. AMGA (2012) *Medical Group Compensation and Financial Survey*. Alexandria, VA: American Medical Group Association.

4. NRMP (2012) *Data Release and Research Committee: Results of the 2012 NRMP Program Director Survey*. Washington, DC: National Resident Matching Program.

5. NRMP (2011) *Charting Outcomes in the Match, 2011*. Washington, DC: National Resident Matching Program.

6. American Association of Neurological Surgeons: Young Neurosurgeons; available from: http://www.aans.org/en/Young%20Neurosurgeons/Medical%20Students.aspx [accessed 2014 June].

Neurology

Natalie Wheeler, MD, JD and Zachary N. London, MD
University of Michigan Medical School, Ann Arbor, MI

Introduction

Neurology is a cerebral specialty that appeals to people who love logic puzzles and problem-solving. A neurologist needs to be able to tease out subtleties of the medical history and physical examination to focus long and complex differentials.

The stereotyped perception of Neurology as a purely diagnostic specialty is largely outdated. The field of neurologic therapeutics has grown dramatically in the last two decades and neurologists must devote a great deal of time to remaining current. For this reason, Neurology programs are looking for candidates with curiosity and intellectual flexibility, as well as a willingness to engage in self-directed learning.

The demand for community-based neurologists is high and continuing to grow. Academic Neurology is a popular choice for graduates interested in research, medical education, and clinical subspecialty neurology. Outpatient positions range from traditional self-employment in a private office to large multispecialty groups to direct employment by hospital systems. There are also growing opportunities for hospital-based subspecialists such as neuro-hospitalists, neuro-intensivists, and vascular neurologists.

Adult Neurology residency is 4 years long, including a Preliminary or Transitional Year in Internal Medicine followed by 3 years of Clinical Neurology training. The Accreditation Council for Graduate Medical Education (ACGME) and the American Board of Psychiatry and Neurology (ABPN) set basic requirements for postgraduate year PGY-1. This internship must include at least 6 months of Internal Medicine, with an additional 2 months of Internal Medicine, Pediatrics, Emergency Medicine, or Family Medicine. The intern year may include up to 2 months of Neurology, though this is not required. Some Neurology programs offer what have been called advanced positions. Residents seeking these positions must apply concurrently and match into an unaffiliated Preliminary medicine or Transitional program. In the past decade, more programs have begun to offer categorical positions. Residents who match into these programs are guaranteed a PGY-1 position at an affiliated hospital.

Applicants must consider a number of factors when deciding whether to apply to advanced programs, categorical programs, or both. One advantage of only applying to categorical programs is a decrease in the total number of interviews. This strategy also avoids the risk of matching into a Neurology program without also matching into an internship. Applicants in fields like Dermatology, Ophthalmology, and Radiation Oncology may provide stiff competition for Preliminary or Transitional positions, especially in certain cities. Another potential advantage of categorical programs is that some provide integrated clinical and/or didactic neurology experiences during intern year, which may facilitate the transition from internship to Neurology training.

Applying to advanced positions also confers additional flexibility for candidates with personal reasons to spend their intern year in a specific location. Furthermore, many highly-regarded programs only offer advanced positions. Remember that the Neurology program from which you graduate is much more important than where you do your internship program.

> **Insider Tip:** When submitting your applications and your rank lists, do not forget about the intern year. If you choose to interview at programs with advanced positions, make sure you apply to an adequate number of Preliminary medicine or Transitional programs, and that these programs provide adequate training in Internal Medicine to fulfill ACGME requirements.

Adult Neurology programs are structured in many different ways. Almost all residency programs include both inpatient and outpatient rotations, but the proportion varies. Many programs "front-load" their PGY-2 schedules with more demanding rotations that have over-night and weekend responsibilities, allowing senior residents to spend more time on clinic or elective rotations. Other programs distribute call responsibilities evenly among all residents in the program.

Owing to ACGME restrictions on long shifts, many programs have created some form of night-float system for overnight coverage of inpatients and consults. Some programs assign home call during which the resident on call may cover multiple hospital locations, whereas other programs have exclusively in-house call responsibilities. Some programs divide call throughout the year, while others consolidate all responsibilities into blocks.

The average Neurology program recruits five or six residents per class, but some take as few as two or as many as 17 residents each year. Residents in small programs may develop closer relationships with colleagues and enjoy more one-on-one attention from faculty members. In larger programs, on the other hand, individuals are less affected when colleagues miss work because of illness, maternity or paternity leave, interviews, or conferences. Good training can be found in a program of any size.

The ability to analyze research methodology and interpret the clinical literature is an important skill. The ACGME requires Neurology residents to participate in research, but the level of involvement needed to fulfill graduation requirements varies significantly among programs. The National Institute of Neurological Disorders and Stroke (NINDS) offers research grants to support intensive neuroscience research by Neurology residents. Residency positions with dedicated research time funded by these R25 grants are available in a handful of academic centers and can be highly competitive placements for prospective clinician-scientists.

> **Insider Tip:** Residency is an intensive training process no matter where you match. Basic program information is available through the ACGME website, but more detailed information about research opportunities, rotation scheduling, and typical call responsibilities is usually available on the websites of each program. If you have specific criteria, find out which programs meet your needs before you apply.

After finishing residency, about 80% of residents choose to complete a 1- or 2-year fellowship. Some fellowships are accredited by licensing institutions, including the ABPN and the United Council for Neurological Subspecialties (UCNS). Fellows completing an accredited fellowship are then eligible for further subspecialty certification, which can increase their competitiveness for certain types of positions.

The ABPN oversees accreditation of fellowships in Brain Injury Medicine, Clinical Neurophysiology (EEG/EMG), Epilepsy, Hospice and Palliative Care, Neurodevelopmental Disabilities, Neuromuscular Medicine, Pain Medicine, Sleep Medicine, And Vascular Neurology. Fellowship positions accredited by the UCNS include Autonomic Disorders, Behavioral Neurology, Clinical Neuromuscular Pathology, Geriatric Neurology, Headache Medicine, Neurorehabilitation, Neurocritical Care, Neuroimaging, and Neuro-oncology. Many centers offer non-accredited fellowships in common subspecialty areas, including Movement Disorders, Neuro-immunology, Neuro-ophthalmology, Neuro-otology, and Sports Neurology.

Fellowship-trained subspecialists remain in high demand for both academic and private practice positions, though a fellowship should not be considered mandatory for future employment.

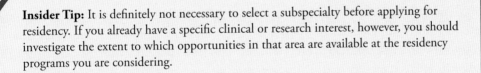

> **Insider Tip:** It is definitely not necessary to select a subspecialty before applying for residency. If you already have a specific clinical or research interest, however, you should investigate the extent to which opportunities in that area are available at the residency programs you are considering.

Preparation

One of the best ways to prepare your residency application is to perform well in your clinical rotations during your third year, particularly in Neurology (if this is a core clinical rotation) and in Internal Medicine.

Most Neurology programs are interested in recruiting residents who have demonstrated commitment to the specialty. Programs may seek candidates who have experience in neuroscience research. Other candidates stand out by participating in community-based organizations relevant to the field of neurology, such as health fairs or subspecialty free clinics. Most schools have a chapter of the Student Interest Group in Neurology (SIGN) affiliated with the

American Academy of Neurology (AAN), the largest neurology professional organization. Being an AAN member will not directly help you get into a residency program, but it can be a great way to network. Membership is often coordinated through the local chapter of SIGN. Student membership in the AAN is free and includes registration for the AAN Annual Meeting. At the Annual Meeting, there are special meetings and events for students and residents, and national leadership opportunities for interested participants. The meeting is a great place to meet residency Program Directors and current residents to discuss career development and residency application in depth. This can be particularly helpful to students whose medical schools provide less direct exposure to the field.

> **Insider Tip:** There are many ways to demonstrate interest in the field of Neurology and in the clinical practice of medicine. While it is important to maintain a good academic performance, research and community service are good ways to show that you are a well-rounded physician.

Many applicants ask about the value of Neurology electives outside of their home institution. If your school is not affiliated with an Academic Neurology Department, an away rotation may be a great way to increase your exposure to the field, solidify your interest in neurology, and obtain a letter of recommendation from an academic neurologist. Some students use an away rotation as a means to connect with faculty whose research or clinical practice is relevant to their interests.

Some students presume an away rotation with a program of interest will boost the chance of matching there. If your performance is stellar, this presumption may prove true, but it is risky. An away rotation requires rapid assimilation of hospital culture, rounding customs, and electronic medical records, all of which may be very different than those of your home school. You will be directly compared to other students who have familiarity with the curriculum, the hospital, and its computer system. The steeper learning curve may impair the visiting student's chances.

Program Directors may view an away rotation as a sign of strong interest and intent to rank that program highly. When a Program Director sees a letter of recommendation (LoR) from someone outside your home institution, they may doubt your level of interest in their program.

> **Insider Tip:** Away rotations have benefits and drawbacks. They can be a great way to increase your experience with the field and may positively influence your application slightly, but they are not necessary for a successful match in Neurology.

Chapter 3

Applying

In 2013, 361 PGY-1 and 331 PGY-2 neurology positions were offered for a total of 692 positions; 361 (52.2%) of these positions were filled by US Seniors and 96.1% of the total positions offered were filled. International Medical Graduates (IMGs) filled 34.1% of the positions. According to data from the 2012 National Resident Matching Program (NRMP®) *Program Director Survey*, the average program receives 374 applications, interviews 55 candidates, and ranks 46 candidates for a class of five residents. In 2011, the mean United States Medical Licensing Examination® (USMLE®) Step 1 and 2 scores of matched US Seniors were 225 and 233, respectively [1–5].

In a recent NRMP survey of Neurology Program Directors, 69% reported that they required a target USMLE Step 1 score for a candidate to receive an interview and 98% indicated that they seldom or never offer interviews to candidates who failed Step 1 on their first attempt.

QUICK FACTS

Rank: Competitive
Average salary: $249 250
Residency years: 4 years (including Internal Medicine internship)
Number of residency positions: 692 (361 PGY-1 and 331 PGY-2)
Number of filled residency positions: 665 (345 PGY-1 and 320 PGY-2)
Number filled by US Seniors: 361 (52.2%)
Number of applicants for PGY-1:
　US Seniors: 374
　Total: 906
Median number of applications:
　US Seniors: 20
　Independent: 50
Median number of interviews offered:
　US Seniors: 15
　Independent: 9
Median number of programs ranked:
　US Seniors: 11
　Independent: 7
Average resident work hours: 50–80 hours
Average attending work hours: 50–60 hours
Resident call: In-house
Data based upon [1–3]

> ✓ **Insider Tip:** If your USMLE Step 1 score or pre-clinical grades are low, consider taking Step 2 to make yourself as competitive as possible.

LoRs are also an important component of the application. In fact, 93% of Program Directors cited LoRs as a factor in determining which applicants to interview, compared with 85% using USMLE Step 1 scores as a major factor. In general, Neurology programs will expect to see at least one letter from a neurologist. Other letters may be obtained from anyone who knows you well, though most students choose Internal Medicine or other medical subspecialties. If you did any significant research during medical school, you may consider including a letter from your research mentor or the Principal Investigator. If you have a PhD in a medical field, a letter from your thesis advisor or faculty mentor is expected.

The personal statement is often dreaded by medical students, but can be a great opportunity to show some personality and let programs get to know you. If necessary, the personal statement can be a chance to explain special circumstances affecting your application. If your personal statement is well written and interesting, it can be a compelling introduction that will favorably influence your interviewers. If your personal statement is incoherent, offensive,

Chapter 3

or poorly written, this will work against you. If English is not your first language, prospective interviewers may use this to gauge your proficiency.

> **Insider Tip:** While letters from senior faculty or prominent researchers are impressive, it is often better to ask for letters from people who know you well. A form letter summarizing your résumé is less meaningful than a more personalized, thoughtful letter from someone less well-known.

Scores and grades may influence which candidates are invited to interview, but the interview day itself is one of the most important factors determining your place on the program's rank list. You will meet several residents and faculty whose role, in part, is to determine how you might fit into the residency program as a whole. Most Program Directors try to assemble a group of interviewers with diverse interests and experiences. Your interview day is your chance to show off the things that make you unique, but remember that you are applying for a professional position. While you should not hesitate to talk about your non-medical interests, the interview is not the time to talk about an argument you had with your significant other or to ask for personal medical advice. You should also assume that everyone you encounter during the interview day may be asked for their impressions of you, so behave accordingly.

> **Insider Tip:** Do not forget that the formal interviews are only part of the evaluation on interview day. Otherwise stellar candidates can drop low on the rank list for bad behavior, such as rudeness to administrative staff or inappropriate comments to residents during the tour. Be polite and gracious to everyone you meet, not just the faculty with whom you interview.

Finally, many candidates have concerns about whether interviewers expect thank you notes after an interview day. While a thank you note should not affect how a program ranks you, not sending one may be taken as a lack of interest. Unless you had a bad experience and do not intend to rank a program, you should send the Program Director an email or hand-written thank you note within about 2 weeks of the interview day. You may also consider sending a note to other interviewers, the Chair, and the Program Coordinator, but these are not absolutely necessary. Make the note as personal as possible. Other interviewers may forward thank you notes to the Program Director, so try to avoid using the same wording in all of them. If you have additional questions after the end of the interview day, you should feel free to email your interviewers or the program coordinator.

Extra Insider Tips:

- **Try not to miss the dinner!** Nearly every program hosts a dinner or other social gathering the evening before the interview day. This is a great opportunity for you to observe informal interactions between the residents and help you decide whether you can see yourself as part of the group. Have fun, but do not forget that the residents are evaluating you. Residents often sit on selection committees and they are not shy about sharing anecdotes about inappropriate behavior.

- **Prepare for the interview in advance!** While an encyclopedic knowledge of the program is not expected, it is helpful to review the program website and ask faculty at your home program for their impressions of institutions where you are interviewing. Mentioning specific features of the program that are of interest to you, when done sincerely, will demonstrate your interest in the program.

- **Keep it real!** Anything you put on your application or bring up during your interview is fair game for questions, including research experiences, language fluency, and extracurricular interests. Most interviewers have at least one or two stories about candidates who wrote about their love of literature, but could not recall the last book they read. If you were only peripherally involved in a research project and do not fully understand it in detail, resist the temptation to exaggerate your level of participation.

- **Ask good questions!** The interview day is not just for the program to learn about you. Figure out what is most important to you, and what you need to know to make an informed decision. In asking questions, try to avoid phrasing that might seem negative or critical. For example, it is reasonable to ask about call schedules and workload, but asking "Do you think the residents here work too hard?" may be off-putting. The same question asked in a slightly different way will get the same information and leave a more positive impression.

- **Consider applying for research grants/fellowships.** There are multiple medical student awards and scholarships offered by the AAN. These include but are not limited to the G. Milton Shy Essay Award (Clinical Neurology), Roland P. Mackey Essay Award (History of Neurology), Saul R. Korey Essay Award (Experimental Neurology), Lawrence C. McHenry Research Award (History of Neurology), Medical Student Essay Award, Medical Student Prize for Excellence, Medical Student Summer Research Scholarship, and Minority Scholars Program.

Chapter 3

References

1. NRMP (2013) *Data Release and Research Committee: Results of the 2013 NRMP Applicant Survey by Preferred Specialty and Applicant Type.* Washington, DC: National Resident Matching Program.

2. NRMP (2013) *Results and Data: 2013 Main Residency Match®.* Washington, DC: National Resident Matching Program.

3. AMGA (2012) *Medical Group Compensation and Financial Survey.* Alexandria, VA: American Medical Group Association.

4. NRMP (2012) *Data Release and Research Committee: Results of the 2012 NRMP Program Director Survey.* Washington, DC: National Resident Matching Program.

5. NRMP (2011) *Charting Outcomes in the Match, 2011.* Washington, DC: National Resident Matching Program.

Obstetrics and Gynecology

Kathleen Dunn, MD, Christine Miller, MD, and D. Yvette LaCoursiere, MD, MPH
UCSD School of Medicine, San Diego, CA

Introduction

Obstetrics and Gynecology is a varied discipline requiring medical, obstetrical, and surgical expertise while caring for women across their lifespan. Obstetrician-gynecologists (OB-GYNs) serve as the primary-care provider for many women. In this role, they have the opportunity to educate patients about a variety of subjects including diet and exercise, contraception, and prenatal care, as well as to follow women from their adolescence through to their golden years. Many OB-GYNs develop strong relationships with their patients due to the ability to foster this kind of continuity. Within the role as the primary health-care provider for women, physicians in this field perform many procedures in addition to surgeries. From IUD placements to cervical biopsies, an OB-GYN must master a variety of skills. Beyond office procedures, OB-GYNs are also skilled surgeons performing a wide range of surgeries including laparotomy, laparoscopy, and robotic approaches for both benign and malignant pathologies.

As a result, the field of Obstetrics and Gynecology often attracts applicants who crave this versatility. Residents cite the ability to do it all without compromise as the reason they chose Obstetrics and Gynecology. Students who are interested in health policy or global health will also find that the field encompasses many topics that pertain to general public health. A successful applicant will be highly accomplished academically and one who can multi-task and work efficiently. Residency programs in Obstetrics and Gynecology aim to recruit students who will thrive in the often-chaotic environment of Labor and Delivery, have the self-discipline to practice and refine their surgical skills, and possess a passion for educating patients.

The Obstetrics and Gynecology residency is 4 years. The vast majority of residencies are categorical ($n = 1237$). Only 22 Preliminary residency positions were available in the United States in 2013. Many residency graduates practice general Obstetrics and Gynecology. However, the discipline offers a wide variety of subspecialties for those who have a penchant for medical or surgical practice, various procedure types, and disease processes.

There are four board certified subspecialties: Gynecology Oncology (46 positions per year), Maternal Fetal Medicine (98 positions), Reproductive Endocrinology and Infertility (45 positions), and Women's Pelvic Medicine and Reconstructive Surgery (51 positions, often called Urogynecology). Though not official boarded subspecialties, additional fellowship training is available in Family Planning (29 positions), Pediatric and Adolescent Gynecology (eight positions), and Minimally Invasive Gynecologic Surgery (67 positions). Additional mentored research programs are available to OB-GYNs (Women's Reproductive Health Research Program).

> **Insider Tip:** Applicants should review the variety of fellowships available after residency, as these options make Obstetrics and Gynecology one of the most versatile residencies.

The 80-hour work week has made the specialty more enticing. Interns in Obstetrics and Gynecology work quite hard. From day 1, most interns participate in procedures and have graded responsibility for patient care as they progress through the milestones. Interns on the oncology and obstetric services often have the longest hours (butting against the 80-hour work week limit) and arrive at the hospital at 5 a.m. After the intern year, the hours tend to improve. Most programs have developed night-float systems to comply with the workweek regulations, a boon to residents, as the days of every third night call are gone. When not on a night-float rotation, residents usually take one weekend call per week and chief residents at some programs have home call. As a procedural specialty, all programs are required to have 24-hour attending coverage in the hospital.

> **Insider Tip:** Do not ask about hours and vacation time at the interview. This information is available online.

Preparation

Many programs emphasize excellence in the third-year clinical clerkships when selecting applicants to interview. Exceptional performance with grades of Honors (or your school's equivalent) in the majority of your clerkships is ideal, especially OB-GYN, Medicine, and Surgery. Additionally, specific comments from your evaluators in the Medical Student Performance Evaluation (MSPE) can round out your picture as an applicant and portray you favorably.

Research is not required, but having a scholarly activity such as a research, community service, or quality improvement project can help set you apart from other applicants. However, at the interview you must be able to describe the work in detail, because applicants who are unable to discuss their project comfortably are suspect.

Pursue your passions during medical school. The endeavors that you enjoy will always come across better to programs than those done just to round out your application. Among the endless activities to pursue are those that demonstrate a commitment to research or service, international work, foreign languages, underserved populations, and education. Think about what each activity meant and how to portray that in your application. Each program is looking for something slightly different. Some are more interested in your research project, while others prefer to see a penchant for service. Also, consider your role in each pursuit. Were you a leader? Part of a team? Or simply a participant? Programs like to see leaders and team players.

Chapter 3

Identify mentors at your medical school who can help guide you through the application process (ideally, someone you have worked with either clinically or on a research project or other endeavor). Your mentors can help you choose programs suited to your interests and competitiveness as an applicant, as well as aid you with your personal statement and application. Having more than one mentor can provide different perspectives of the process.

Applying

In 2013, 1259 Obstetrics and Gynecology positions were offered at the PGY-1 level; 76.6% of these positions were filled by US Seniors and 99.1% of the total positions offered were filled. International Medical Graduates (IMGs) filled 12.2% of the positions. According to data from the 2012 National Resident Matching Program (NRMP®) *Program Director Survey*, the average program receives 370 applications, interviews 66 candidates, and ranks 56 candidates for a class of five residents [1–5].

The best resource for learning about residency programs nationwide is the Association of Professors of Gynecology and Obstetrics (APGO) website (https://www.apgo.org/student/residency.html), which hosts an APGO Residency Directory that sorts residency programs by state, institu-

tion, and size. It contains a wealth of specific information on each program that is valuable to guide your program selection and in preparation for each interview. This site also lists mean United States Medical Licensing Examination® (USMLE®) scores of the residents in their programs and can be used to gauge their competitiveness.

QUICK FACTS

Rank: Competitive
Median salary: $303 350
Residency years: 4 years (including Preliminary)
Number of residency positions: 1259 (75.0%)
Number of filled residency positions: 1248 (99.1%)
Number filled by US Seniors: 944 (74.8%)
Number of applicants:
  US Seniors: 1059
  Total: 1783
Ratio of applicants to available residency positions: 1.4:1
Median number of applications:
  US Seniors: 30
  Independent: 47
Median number of interviews offered:
  US Seniors: 16
  Independent: 12
Median number of programs ranked:
  US Seniors: 11
  Independent: 9
Average resident work hours: 80 hours
Average attending work hours: 80 hours
Data based upon [1–3]

Insider Tip: Meet with faculty and review the APGO residency site to identify potential programs. Always select several "reach" and "safety-net" programs and aim to interview at 10–12 places.

Many top-tier programs use board scores and/or number of honors in the clinical years to screen applicants. They often use the step 1 score as a screening criterion, often employing the national mean. Applicants with USMLE Step 1 scores below the national mean may be granted an interview if their Step 2 scores are markedly higher. Scores of 240 and above are often needed to be competitive at the top-tier programs. In 2011, the mean USMLE Step 1 and 2 scores of matched US Seniors were 220 and 233, respectively.

As you compile your application and prepare for interview season, consider the impression you want someone to have of you after finishing reading your application. Try to create a theme to weave throughout your application and interview. What is your passion? Is it research, medical education, or international work? For example, an applicant interested in international work in South or Central America may emphasize Spanish language skills as an interpreter, commitment to the underserved Latino population domestically, and a research project abroad in Honduras. Though these are all separate projects, the same theme translates throughout. Whatever your niche is, be sure to portray it.

> **Insider Tip:** Make sure your entire application is completely free of spelling or grammatical errors.

Your personal statement can be a great way to draw everything together. It is also an opportunity for you to tell the programs something that may not have been apparent elsewhere in your application. Aim to tell a good story and grab your reader from the beginning, but stay away from anything strange. You do not want someone to remember your personal statement because it was "the weird one." Make sure you edit it thoroughly for spelling and grammatical errors. Have your mentors, advisers, and classmates review it, as well as people outside of medicine who might offer a fresh perspective.

> **Insider Tip:** The Electronic Residency Application Service (ERAS®) has a Hobbies and Interests section that can be a great opportunity to list some unique things that will certainly be talking points during interviews. Do you run marathons? Brew your own beer? Were you a competitive Irish Dancer? This is the spot for those fun facts.

Letters of recommendation should be from faculty members who know you well. At least one should be from an Obstetrics and Gynecology faculty member at your medical school. Some of the letter writers should be familiar with your performance during your clinical rotations.

> **Insider Tip:** If you do not receive an interview at a program you are seriously considering, your faculty may be able to help you, but it still might not be enough to place you in a position to match. If you have a strong reason to be at that program, ask your faculty for assistance.

Chapter 3

Be yourself. The most important part of the interview is to find a program that suits you. While it is of the utmost importance to be professional and respectful, you want to portray yourself as honestly as possible. It is better to know that a program is not the right "fit" at the interview than after you match there. Dinners and lunches can be important, as they portray the overall feel or tone of the program. If a dinner is hosted and no faculty or staff attend, that may tell you something. Many programs consider the input of faculty, staff, and residents. Remember that everything you do or say is fair game at your interviews. Several capable applicants have been removed from the rank list for treating staff disrespectfully. Use the APGO Residency Directory to obtain basic program information and reference it in your interviews. Showing the interviewers that you have thoughtfully considered the program and done your homework is important. The internet can be used to identify a great deal of preliminary information about a program. Availability of information on the internet can be a two-edged sword. Remember that information on blogs about programs can be biased by those who take the time to write them and your personal information may be available on social media sites.

Insider Tip: Erase or lock your social media sites, or at least make certain that they portray you in a positive light.

"Second looks" are not required; indeed, rank lists may often be complete prior to your arrival. If not inconvenient or excessively costly, and you feel the visit would aid your decision, going for a second look is reasonable. However, it is usually not sufficient to sway an applicant's position on a rank list.

Extra Insider Tip:
- **Consider applying for research grants/fellowships.** One award specific to the field is the John Gibbons Medical Student Travel Award offered by the American Congress of Obstetricians and Gynecologists.

References

1. NRMP (2013) *Data Release and Research Committee: Results of the 2013 NRMP Applicant Survey by Preferred Specialty and Applicant Type.* Washington, DC: National Resident Matching Program.
2. NRMP (2013) *Results and Data: 2013 Main Residency Match®.* Washington, DC: National Resident Matching Program.
3. AMGA (2012) *Medical Group Compensation and Financial Survey.* Alexandria, VA: American Medical Group Association.
4. NRMP (2012) *Data Release and Research Committee: Results of the 2012 NRMP Program Director Survey.* Washington, DC: National Resident Matching Program.
5. NRMP (2011) *Charting Outcomes in the Match, 2011.* Washington, DC: National Resident Matching Program.

Ophthalmology

Kian Eftekhari, MD and Paul J. Tapino, MD
Scheie Eye Institute, Perelman School of Medicine, University of Pennsylvania Medical School, Philadelphia, PA

Introduction

Ophthalmology is a primarily office-based surgical subspecialty that uses a wide variety of technologies and techniques to treat eye disease. Ophthalmologists have to be visual learners and rely on pattern recognition to diagnose and treat diseases of the cornea, lens, and retina. In addition, they utilize microsurgical techniques to remove cataracts or operate on the retina. The specialty demands the ability to think on your feet to treat eye problems on an everyday basis, but also demands an interest in performing procedures. Most patients are seen in an outpatient setting rather than in the hospital. The specialty is competitive due to the manageable hours compared to other surgical fields and reasonable salary. Matching in Ophthalmology generally demands a strong application with some research.

Ophthalmologists usually work in an academic setting or in private practice, often as part of an Ophthalmology multispecialty group rather than working for a hospital. Most comprehensive ophthalmologists see patients in clinic 3–4 days a week and operate 1–2 days per week. Comprehensive ophthalmologists perform mainly cataract surgery. Among the many subspecialties within Ophthalmology are Cornea, Glaucoma, Vitreo-retinal Surgery, Oculoplastic Surgery, Uveitis, Neuro-ophthalmology, Pediatric Ophthalmology, and Ophthalmic Pathology. A comprehensive ophthalmologist in an academic setting may see 30–40 patients per day, while in private practice an ophthalmologist might see upwards of 50 patients daily.

Job satisfaction among ophthalmologists is among the highest within medicine. Many people choose to do Ophthalmology because it affords the opportunity to develop long-term relationships with patients and treat medical conditions while also being a surgical subspecialty. Medical students not interested in doing procedures probably would not be a good fit for Ophthalmology, although some providers do not perform surgery on a routine basis.

Residency is 4 years long, including a Preliminary or Transitional Year. Many ophthalmology residents choose to do a Transitional Year, as it affords the ability to take care of medical and surgical patients. Ophthalmology residency has the advantage of being fairly structured and relatively uniform across different programs in the country. Typically, the first year of Ophthalmology residency (PGY-2) is focused on learning examination techniques, building a knowledge base, and gaining some exposure to the Operating Room. The second year of residency usually involves a heavier clinical load, more time doing surgery, and often the heaviest call schedule. At most programs, the third year of residency is mainly devoted to learning cataract surgery. The national residency review committee requires at least 86 cataract procedures as Primary Surgeon over the course of residency, although most programs exceed this number and generally average at least 155 cataract cases. However, while it may be tempting to think that a higher volume of surgical cases indicates a better program, this depends on career plans after residency. Most Ophthalmology residents go on to complete a fellowship and in many cases this may mean one does not perform cataract surgery for the rest of your career. Therefore, if a medical student is interested in doing retina surgery, it may not be as meaningful to go to a program with high cataract surgery numbers if the retina department is not as strong. It is best to consider programs that are strong in a number of specialties and provide adequate surgical numbers across different fields, such as oculoplastics, pediatrics, and retina.

Insider Tip: Many residency programs also have fellowship programs. While this is not necessarily bad, as fellows contribute to resident education, having a large number of fellows – especially cornea fellows who will want to perform cataract surgery – can have a negative impact on resident surgical volume.

Call responsibilities vary among programs, with the most intensive call generally during PGY-2. However, some programs (like ours) have more intensive call during PGY-3, when the resident has a much higher knowledge base and is more efficient. Very few Ophthalmology programs have in-house call. The majority of programs have home call, but depending on the number of hospitals or trauma centers they cover, there may be numerous consults in the middle of the night. As Ophthalmology is a specialty where general practitioners may not be able to do a majority of the clinical exam, it often is necessary to come into the hospital to see a consult just to make a diagnosis, even if it is not truly emergent.

Insider Tip: While call duties are one consideration when choosing a residency, Ophthalmology is generally a less intensive field than other surgical subspecialties, so that judging a program by its call schedule may be less important than other factors.

Programs vary in the facilities they offer residents, but one thing to look for is a Veterans Administration (VA) hospital at the program. While this is not a requirement to ensure you will meet the surgical numbers, in many cases VA hospitals are where residents perform a high volume of cataract surgery.

Insider Tip: The presence of a VA hospital in an Ophthalmology program usually is a good sign that the program has adequate clinical and surgical volume.

Chapter 3

Preparation

Performing well during medical school, especially on the Medicine and Surgery clinical rotations, is the surest way to match into Ophthalmology. Many medical schools also have an Ophthalmology rotation and, while performing well is important, the evaluation you get may not be as important, as these rotations are in general more lenient than the core clerkships. Performance on an Ophthalmology rotation may be better reflected in the quality of a letter of recommendation (LoR) than on the clerkship grade.

> **Insider Tip:** LoRs are very important in Ophthalmology. It is a small field, so that many people at different programs know each other personally. Having your personality and work ethic shine through on a LoR can be a key factor in getting an interview.

It is very common for medical students to discover an interest in Ophthalmology on elective rotations later in medical school. While it is most noteworthy to get involved in research activities at an early stage, pursuing other activities during medical school is also valuable. For example, participating in student groups and serving in a leadership position is important. Research is also important, especially if you are looking to match in an academic program. In many Ophthalmology programs, the clinical faculty who educate the residents are actually in private practice. Therefore, research may be less important in these settings. Nevertheless, demonstrating an interest in research can only help your application. Even if you do a project in another field before you developed an interest in Ophthalmology, this can at least indicate an interest in research.

If you are considering taking a year off to do research, there are Doris Duke and National Eye Institute fellowships at some academic medical centers that focus on Ophthalmology research. These typically occur between the third and fourth years of medical school. If you pursue one of these programs, be prepared to talk about it on interviews.

Many medical schools have an Ophthalmology rotation available to their students. If not, or if you would like to match in a specific area of the country, consider doing an away elective. We do not routinely encourage our medical students to do away electives, because they may do more harm than good for your application. If you have a strong application and are not focused on a specific geographic area where you would like to match, there is often no need to do an away elective. Your Medical Student Dean or Ophthalmology Student Coordinator may be able to take a look at your application and tell you whether it is competitive. If you do an away rotation, it can be high risk, high reward. If you are trying so hard to make a good impression that you appear too intense or over-eager, it could doom your application to that specific residency. We have had medical students who, while clearly very smart and hard-working, were just a little too aggressive and did not make the right impression. On the other hand, if you perform well and get to know a few faculty, it can certainly bolster your chances of matching into that program. Away electives are commonplace in Ophthalmology, but just be certain that you understand the risks as well. If you do an away elective, make sure to try to obtain a letter of recommendation from a faculty member at that institution.

Another way to distinguish your application is to present a poster at the American Academy of Ophthalmology (AAO) or Association of University Professors in Ophthalmology (AUPO) meetings. The former is the main society meeting, while the latter attracts mainly Program Directors and Department Chairs, and is a good networking opportunity.

Applying

In 2013, there were 583 applicants for 460 Ophthalmology positions offered, all but five of which were filled (applicant match rate of 78%); 96% of the matched applicants were US graduates and 4% were foreign graduates. Between 2003 to 2013, the matched rate has slightly increased (from 67 to 78%) [1, 2].

United States Medical Licensing Examination® (USMLE®) Step 1 is often a factor that gives Program Directors a first cut of medical students whom they would like to interview. In 2013, the average USMLE Step 1 score for students who matched in ophthalmology was 239, while the number for students who did not match was 222. For the sake of comparison, 10 years previously these numbers were 228 and 208, respectively. While many programs accept medical students with lower scores, it will make it harder to get interviews unless your LoRs or another aspect of your application is outstanding. If you are not happy with your USMLE Step 1 score, consider taking Step 2 early enough so that it can be put on your application.

In Ophthalmology, LoRs are a key aspect of the application. Many well-known faculty around the country write letters for numerous medical students, but it is more important to get a quality letter from somebody who knows you well than a generic letter from a famous ophthalmologist. Program Directors around the country receive these generic letters all the time and if yours is not significantly better or more insightful than the other letters they have received from the same person, it may not carry much weight. If possible, you should obtain two letters from Ophthalmology faculty and one from a non-ophthalmologist or research mentor. In addition, you may want to obtain a fourth letter from any faculty member because some Preliminary programs may require it.

For Ophthalmology, the application process is coordinated by SF Match (San Francisco Matching Program; www.SFmatch.org), which is an entity with its own timeline that differs from that for Electronic Residency Application Service (ERAS®), which coordinates most other residency matches, including the one for your Preliminary Year. Therefore, you will have to

QUICK FACTS

Rank: Highly competitive
Average salary: $371 987
Residency years: 4 years (including Preliminary)
Number of residency positions: 460
Number of filled residency positions: 455 (98.9%)
Number filled by US Seniors: 411 (89.3%)
Number of applicants: 583
Match rate: 78%
Average number of applications: 58
Average resident work hours: 50–70 hours
Average attending work hours: 40–60 hours
Resident call: Program-dependent
Data based upon [1, 2]

apply to both, but the Ophthalmology application is due earlier. There is not a firm deadline for the SF Match applications, but in general you should try to submit your completed application with LoRs before Labor Day so that it is reviewed in the first batch. Interviews may occur as early as late September or early October, but most take place in November and December. The interview schedule is fast and furious, and many programs use the same weekends for interviews each year. In general, it is good to have a rough idea of your rank list before interviews so that if there are scheduling conflicts between programs, you know which one you would like to pick. Be prepared to respond quickly for available interview dates as these will fill up! The best thing you can do is have a calendar available and use an email address that you can check on your mobile device. Some programs even call you directly to invite you for an interview, so be prepared. Be courteous to the administrative assistant or program administrator with whom you speak; that person often plays an integral role in the process, though does not make the final decisions.

The interview is a very important factor in your future position on the rank list. Residency programs usually compile their rank list the same day as the interview and then collate the lists from all interview days. If you have a faculty member advocating for you who knows someone at a program you are visiting, you can try to have them call beforehand to put in a good word. However, if you have a faculty member call to tell a program you are ranking them highly, you can only do this for one program. On the interview day, be yourself, stay positive, and try to act professionally. Remember, interviewers are evaluating what kind of colleague you will make, so even if the residents are casual do not let down your guard too much. There often is a dinner before or after the interview, and these events offer a more casual setting for asking residents questions about the program and getting to know them better. Remember, Ophthalmology is a small field, so even if you do not anticipate ranking a program highly, always try to make a good impression, because you will likely run into your co-applicants and residents in that program in the future.

Extra Insider Tip:
- **Consider applying for research grants/fellowships.** One award specific to the field is the RBP Medical Student Fellowship supported by the Research to Prevent Blindness Grant Program.

References

1. AMGA (2012) *Medical Group Compensation and Financial Survey*. Alexandria, VA: American Medical Group Association.
2. SF Match; available from: https://www.sfmatch.org/SpecialtyInsideAll.aspx?id=6&typ=2&name=Ophthalmology [accessed September 2014].

Orthopedic Surgery

George S. M. Dyer, MD
Harvard Combined Orthopaedic Residency Program, Harvard Medical School, Boston, MA

Introduction

Orthopedic surgeons are trained in the surgical and non-surgical management of musculo-skeletal disease, injury, and congenital disease. Orthopedics is fundamentally a branch of Surgery, although the training has become so specialized that only a fraction of the first year of training is spent doing General Surgery. It is an anatomically-based, interventional discipline, requiring both technical mastery and also cognitive understanding. It is a growing field with fast-moving frontiers. Therefore, Orthopedic residency programs are looking for strong students with demonstrated interest in surgery and research. As it has become a highly sought-after field, Orthopedics attracts some of the strongest and most motivated applicants in any branch of medicine.

The caricature of an orthopedic surgeon is a physically large, inexpressive, former athlete interested only in broken bones. In fact there are many subspecialties within Orthopedics and careers can be as varied as the physicians who choose them. There are at least nine recognized subspecialties:

- Orthopedic Trauma
- Joint Reconstruction (Arthroplasty)
- Spine
- Sports
- Shoulder/Elbow

- Hand/Upper Extremity
- Orthopedic Oncology
- Pediatric Orthopedics
- Foot and Ankle

Some surgeons tailor their practice of Orthopedics in ways that make it physically demanding. For example, some complex operations on the spine can last 10 hours or more. Some surgeons who are based in academic medical centers have practices built around research and innovation. Others craft practices that are much more predictable and less exhausting, emphasizing quick outpatient or office-based procedures. Orthopedic Surgery offers great flexibility in shaping a career that is right for you.

Orthopedic residency is 5 years long. Although the internship was once a separate year of General Surgery as a Preliminary to detailed orthopedic training, it is now all a single process and almost always carried out together in one place. The intern year is about 50% General Surgery and 50% Orthopedics. All 5 years are based in a hospital setting, although portions will take place in outpatient clinics or ambulatory surgery centers. Almost all residents take an additional year of fellowship in one of the subspecialties listed above and in recent years many residents have done more than one fellowship. This makes the full duration of training 6 or 7 years after medical school.

Generally speaking, Orthopedic Surgery residents work pretty hard. Although their work schedules are limited to 80 hours per week, most junior residents (interns and PGY-2) work close to that. The exact pattern and order of different rotations varies from program to program, but all surgical training works on the principle of *graduated responsibility*. The intern year is largely spent learning to be a doctor and to think like a surgeon, while managing patients before and after surgery, and to mastering the fundamental tools of surgical technique like using a scalpel and suturing. As the years progress, residents spend more time learning to perform more complex orthopedic operations and managing orthopedic problems in the Emergency Department. In the final years, residents take nearly full responsibility for planning and performing operations, under the supervision of the attending staff.

The training for all the surgical disciplines is longer than for non-surgical ones, because the technical skills of surgery take time to develop and they are not really taught in medical school. Orthopedic surgical training in particular can be demanding because much of it is based in busy hospitals and it follows the unpredictable rhythms of trauma, surgical complications, and other emergencies. However, after training, an orthopedic surgeon enjoys a much wider choice of lifestyle and schedule.

> **Insider Tip:** Do not rule out a career in Orthopedic Surgery because residency seems too hard. That is only 5 or 6 years out of a career.

Preparation

Pre-Clinical Years

Excellent performance throughout medical school is important, starting in the pre-clinical years. There is also no better way to study for United States Medical Licensing Examination® (USMLE®) Step 1 than by paying careful attention during the first 2 years of medical school.

This is also a great time to explore orthopedic research. Seek out an orthopedic advisor from among the hospital's clinical faculty. If you are not sure where to start, ask for help from the Student Affairs Office or Academic Dean. You will be surprised how welcoming most orthopedic research faculty are. The earlier you present yourself, the easier it is to incorporate you into an existing project or to help you to design one of your own.

> **Insider Tip:** If you are reading this during your third or even fourth year, having just discovered an interest in Orthopedics, do not despair! It is not essential to have 10 orthopedic publications by the time you apply. If you have completed other serious scholarship during medical school, that will be good enough. We are just interested in gauging your brains, your creativity, and your stamina for seeing a project to its finish.

Clinical Years

During your clinical years, give your all in every rotation. No doubt your evaluations in Surgery and Orthopedic subinternships will be considered strongly, but you may safely assume that almost all successful applicants will have earned honors in those rotations. Do not overlook the importance of Medicine, Obstetrics and Gynecology, and Pediatrics in your overall portfolio.

> **Insider Tip:** Some programs quietly place particular emphasis on "sleeper" rotations like Psychiatry or Family Medicine to try to discern candidates who work hard all the time from ones who pick and choose where to make an honest effort. Think of it as a litmus test of your work ethic. We want to know how carefully you work when you think no one is watching.

During our residency admissions committee meetings, the faculty may disagree about many facets of different applicants. Does Alpha Omega Alpha really matter if you aced USMLE Step 1? Is a strong letter from another discipline like Neurology or General Surgery worth as much as one from an orthopedic surgeon? In the end, most of those things end as a toss-up. No one of those factors will ever spell the difference between matching or not.

But there is one thing we all agree on: *nobody likes a gunner.* Be nice to the other subinterns on your rotations. Help them out and try to make them look good – I promise you that kind of thing gets noticed. On the other hand, if a student earns a reputation for taking advantage of his teammates or stabbing them in the back, he/she is doomed.

Although individual accomplishment is important, remember that "surgery is a team sport." It is mostly a distracting cliché that orthopedic surgeons are all ex-athletes. Yet within that stereotype is a useful kernel of truth. When we hire a resident we are, essentially, signing a medical student to a 5-year playing contract on a team where the lives of our patients hang in the balance.

> **Insider Tip:** Make sure your every action in the hospital demonstrates that you are the kind of person we want on our team. Be reliable. Be truthful. Put the interests of your teammates above your own and put the interest of your patients above everything.

Applying

In its annual statistical report, the National Resident Matching Program (NRMP®) reported that in 2013, Orthopedic Surgery had 163 accredited programs, offering 693 positions to start training at the PGY-1 level. There were 833 US Senior applicants and 205 other applicants (total = 1038). That works out to 1.5 applicants for every position. After Match Day, 636 US Seniors were matched (76%) and a total of 692 out of 693 positions were filled (99.9%). International Medical Graduates (IMGs) filled 2.2% of the total positions. According to data from the 2012 NRMP *Program Director Survey*, the average program receives 530 applications, interviews 62 candidates, and ranks 51 candidates for a class of five residents [1–6].

A publication of the American Academy of Orthopaedic Surgeons reports that successful applicants had an average USMLE score of 230, 32% were Alpha Omega Alpha, 62% had publications, and 93% had worked on prior research projects. Orthopedics is undoubtedly a competitive field. It may be helpful to consider some common questions and answers as a way to explore this issue further.

- **My USMLE Step 1 score was 220. Should I just give up?** No. Do not write yourself off. But understand that, fair or not, that number carries a great deal of meaning, especially early in the application review process. Many programs use a cut off USMLE Step 1 score to help filter the many hundreds of applications they receive. For example, our institution receives more than 700 applications each year for 12 positions. Although we have no absolute cut off number, we are less likely to seriously consider applicants with scores below 220. In 2011, the mean USMLE Step 1 and 2 scores of matched US Seniors nationally were 240 and 245, respectively. Foreign medical graduates and applicants who failed to match in a previous year are also considered only on an exceptional basis.

  If you are in any of these positions, you will need to make a big, positive impression in some other way. Consider taking an additional year and delving deeply into a research project. Find an orthopedic mentor and ask for honest advice about how to improve your own candidacy. But do not let that urgency turn you into a lunatic. See the advice above about back-stabbing and gunners.

- **I did much better on USMLE Step 2: will that make up for my low Step 1 score?** No. Again, fair or not, USMLE Step 1 has become the accepted filter; unless the scores are dramatically different, Step 2 does not matter.

- **How many programs should I apply to?** The prevailing wisdom has become that strong students should apply to 35 or more, and weaker ones to more than 50. To really know whether that makes a difference, you would need to know something about successful versus unsuccessful applicants, the number of programs they applied to, and their rankings of the programs where they matched, but this is not available. For what it is worth, the NRMP does release the inverse statistic – in 2013, US Orthopedics programs needed to rank an average of 4.7 applicants per position they wished to fill.

QUICK FACTS

Rank: Highly competitive
Median salary: $515 759
Residency years: 5 years (including Preliminary)
Number of residency positions: 693
Number of filled residency positions: 692 (99.9%)
Number filled by US Seniors: 636 (91.8%)
Number of applicants:
　US Seniors: 833
　Total: 1038
Ratio of applicants to available residency positions: 1.5:1
Median number of applications:
　US Seniors: 62
　Independent: 60
Median number of interviews offered:
　US Seniors: 16
　Independent: 7
Median number of programs ranked:
　US Seniors: 12
　Independent: 6
Average resident work hours: 80 hours
Average attending work hours: 60–70 hours
Resident call: In-house
Data based upon [1–3]

Chapter 3

Interviews

This is probably the most important part of the application process, since scores, grades, and papers only get you an interview. At the interview itself is where we learn whether you are a person with whom we want to live for 5 years – a person we will be proud to call our graduate.

Different residencies have experimented with a myriad ways of figuring this out. Some have very conventional one-on-one or two-on-one conversations. Others have a single large panel that sees every applicant and asks the same questions of them all. Some interviews are deliberately stressful, but most are not.

Try to relax and enjoy the opportunity to speak with your future colleagues. Remember that although you do not want to seem rude or presumptuous, you are there to interview the program as much as the other way around. Think of good questions beforehand and ask them in a polite way.

Insider Tip: Remember that the entire time you are visiting a program you are "on-camera," not just during your official interviews. On interview day, we always ask the residents to report strange or unpleasant personal interactions with applicants, at lunch or during the hospital tour.

References

1. NRMP (2013) *Data Release and Research Committee: Results of the 2013 NRMP Applicant Survey by Preferred Specialty and Applicant Type*. Washington, DC: National Resident Matching Program.
2. NRMP (2013) *Results and Data: 2013 Main Residency Match®*. Washington, DC: National Resident Matching Program.
3. AMGA (2012) *Medical Group Compensation and Financial Survey*. Alexandria, VA: American Medical Group Association.
4. NRMP (2012) *Data Release and Research Committee: Results of the 2012 NRMP Program Director Survey*. Washington, DC: National Resident Matching Program.
5. NRMP (2011) *Charting Outcomes in the Match, 2011*. Washington, DC: National Resident Matching Program.
6. AAOS (2011) *How to Obtain an Orthopaedic Surgery Residency*. Chicago, IL: American Academy of Orthopaedic Surgeons.

Otolaryngology

Benjamin L. Judson, MD, Boris Paskhover, MD, and Elias M. Michaelides, MD
Yale School of Medicine, New Haven, CT

Introduction

Otolaryngology is a diverse surgical subspecialty with a broad scope of practice in terms of patients, diseases, and surgeries. Otolaryngologists care for patients from neonates to geriatrics. They diagnose and manage diseases of the ears, nose, sinuses, larynx, throat, and structures of the face and neck. They generally perform a large number of office procedures but their practice can also include large, lengthy, and complex surgeries. In additional to the practice of General Otolaryngology, specialization through fellowship training after residency is possible in areas such as Head and Neck Surgery, Rhinology/Endoscopic Skull Base Surgery, Sleep Medicine, Otology/Neurotology, Facial Plastics and Reconstructive Surgery, Pediatric Otolaryngology, and Laryngology. Although less common, practitioners can also focus on Otolaryngologic Allergy and Immunology and Geriatric Otolaryngology. Otolaryngologists often interact and at times work closely with a number of other specialists on problems such as head and neck cancers, disorders affecting the vestibular and auditory systems, diseases affecting the airway, voice, and swallowing, facial cosmetic and reconstructive problems, pediatric diseases, and skull base tumors. While general Otolaryngology includes adult and pediatric patients, some otolaryngologists specialize in the care of pediatric patients, including the very youngest, as well as more complex problems in this population.

Otolaryngology is one of the earliest surgical specialties, as evidenced by hospitals such as the London Infirmary for Curing Disease of the Eye and Ear that dates back to 1805. The complexity and importance of the anatomy and systems encountered by otolaryngologists in hearing, speech, breathing, and swallowing, as well as the aesthetic importance of the face, head, and neck, have been associated with intensive technological aspects to practice as well as innovation. Recent advances have included minimally invasive approaches such as transoral robotic surgery, endoscopic sinus surgery, sialoendoscopy, endoscopic otologic procedures, and endoscopic skull base surgery.

Otolaryngology requires precise and delicate surgical skills and a broad knowledge of pathology and physiology. Although Otolaryngology is primarily a surgical field, there is no "medical" counterpart, so that practitioners are the overall expert for diseases in this area. Consequently, they have the opportunity to balance both surgical and medical treatments as components of their practice.

This interesting clinical diversity, flexibility in type of clinical practice, and a competitive salary make otolaryngology residency spots very sought-after. There are just under 300 open residency positions annually and approximately 400 applicants from US medical schools. This means that about a quarter of US graduates applying to Otolaryngology go unmatched each year. As with other competitive surgical subspecialties, Otolaryngology residency programs are looking for students with an accomplished academic background such as membership in Alpha Omega Alpha, high board scores, strong character traits, and research experience and productivity.

There are 107 residency programs in the country, ranging from one to five positions at each postgraduate year level of training. Programs vary in terms of size, geography, greater or lesser academic focus, diverse presence in the different subspecialty areas, and different program cultures. Even with this variation, excellent otolaryngologic training is attainable at the majority of programs.

Insider Tip: Consider major changes within a program. Transitions such as a new Chair, which often come with additional faculty, can result in rapid program growth. The intimate nature of training and relatively small size of most programs means that loss of faculty also has the potential to adversely impact training.

Residency is most often 5 years in duration, including an integrated internship. The intern year consists of General Surgery rotations, 1 month each of Anesthesia, Neurological Surgery, and Emergency Medicine, and up to 3 months of Otolaryngology. The remaining 4 years of residency are spent entirely on Otolaryngology training. A well-rounded residency program will provide access to each of the core subspecialties, as well as good general training. A significant proportion of residents, especially those interested in an academic career, continue on for fellowship (typically for 1 or 2 years) in a subspecialty. In recent years, about half of graduate otolaryngologists have entered fellowship programs.

Being a surgical field means that surgical call starts as an intern. These calls are restricted by Accreditation Council for Graduate Medical Education (ACGME) time limits. Once the first otolaryngology year begins (PGY-2), residents begin taking Otolaryngology call on their own, with higher-level residents and attendings available for support. Some programs institute home call versus in-house call, with differences among programs regarding call responsibilities. By PGY-4 and PGY-5, residents in most programs are considered senior residents and often help support the junior residents or serve as needed for operative coverage.

Insider Tip: Consider how many other programs are in the geographic vicinity and the program volume. Case numbers and exposure to unusual cases depend on the catchment area and population base served by a program.

Call can be a stressful experience, especially when covering airway emergencies and maxillofacial trauma. A resident may be expected to appropriately initially manage life-threatening emergencies such as penetrating neck trauma, airway emergencies such as tracheostomy dislodgement and need for operative airway intervention, carotid blowouts, pediatric airway foreign body aspirations, epiglottitis, recalcitrant epistaxis, orbital hematoma, and orbital entrapment. Your level of exposure to these conditions during residency, combined with an appropriate level of both support and independence, prepares you for your career and enables safe, confident, and appropriate care to patients.

> **Insider Tip:** "Breadth and depth" are terms you may hear about during interviews. This refers to a program's coverage of subspecialty areas, exposure to otolaryngologic patients, and operative case numbers.

Preparation

As in all competitive fields, academic strength is a must, but is only one piece of the puzzle. A strong applicant also demonstrates commitment to Otolaryngology through research and exposure to the field. An applicant who has not shown commitment to Otolaryngology is a risk to the program, since they have not fully explored the field and may be more liable to be unhappy with the specialty they have selected and/or even leave the program.

Letters of recommendation (LoR) and research interest carry significant weight in pre-interview screening as well as the selection process. Obtaining strong LoRs from your home institution is a must for all applicants. If your home program does not have an academic department with residents, all is not lost, since a strong genuine letter still carries weight. Applicants in this situation are encouraged to also do away rotations to help obtain LoRs from some well-known otolaryngologists. The Otolaryngology community can feel surprisingly small at times, in part because of the level of collegiality within the field. This means that someone at the program to which you are applying probably knows the author of your LoRs. In addition to the nature of the letter itself, having a LoR from someone well-known can be helpful.

> **Insider Tip:** Most applicants will have strong academic records. To help catch the eyes of Program Directors, try to show strong character traits through accomplishments and interests, on top of having strong LoRs and research.

Research is an integral part of the field, and there are some 6- to 7-year otolaryngology residency positions that incorporate a 1- to 2-year research component. Applicants are not required to have published multiple articles by the time they apply, but interest and involvement in otolaryngologic research is a must and publications can be helpful.

> **Insider Tip:** Have at least one research topic to be able to discuss in detail on interviews, even if has not been published yet. This demonstrates your understanding of the project and of how to perform successful research.

Chapter 3

Fourth-year rotations at outside programs are more than just a way to get LoRs. You should pick one or two subinternships, if possible. These rotations will solidify your understanding of the field, make you conversational in topics you may be discussing during interviews, and most importantly give the faculty the ability to evaluate you first-hand. Think of these rotations as month-long interviews. Remember that the residents also will be evaluating you to ensure you would be a good addition to their team. If really impressed with your work, residents certainly will pass this information on to the faculty. It may be helpful for you to ask your local faculty to give you advice on which programs you should consider applying for these subinternships.

Insider Tip: How an applicant would "fit" in a program can be an important factor when candidates are ranked. This relates to how an applicant would work interpersonally with the residents and staff.

Applying

In 2013, 292 Otolaryngology positions were offered at the PGY-1 level (US otolaryngology residencies have integrated intern training); 94.5% of these positions were filled by US Seniors and 99.3% of the total positions offered were filled. Two positions were unmatched initially, but these were quickly filled. Seven positions went to US graduates who had gone unmatched from previous years. Six positions were taken by International Medical Graduates (IMGs). With only 292 positions, Otolaryngology comprised only 1.1% of all residency positions in the 2013 match. According to data from the 2012 National Resident Matching Program (NRMP®) *Program Director Survey*, the average program receives 251 applications, interviews 38 candidates, and ranks 32 candidates for a class of three residents [1–5].

QUICK FACTS

Rank: Highly competitive
Median salary: $374 387
Residency years: 5 years (including Intern year)
Number of residency positions: 292
Number of filled residency positions: 290 (99.3%)
Number filled by US graduates: 276 (94.5%)
Number of applicants:
  US Seniors: 387
  Total: 442
Ratio of applicants to available positions: 1.5:1
Median number of applications:
  US Seniors: 56
  Independent: 89
Median number of interviews offered:
  US Seniors: 15
  Independent: 4
Median number of programs ranked:
  US Seniors: 11
  Independent: 4
Average resident work hours: 80 hours
Average attending work hours: 60–70 hours
Resident call: Program-dependent
Data based upon [1–3]

As mentioned previously, academic strength is just one piece of the puzzle, albeit a critical one for applicants. In addition to medical school grades, Alpha Omega Alpha status is one indicator of academic accomplishment. Although not necessary, this can be a helpful honor during the review process. United States Medical Licensing Examination®

(USMLE®) scores are another indicator used by programs, particularly while selecting applicants for interviews. Programs may screen or stratify applications by USMLE board scores prior to more careful review. Although there is no absolute USMLE score required, a lower score may make getting interviews more difficult. High USMLE scores are common among successful applicants, with a significant number of applicants in the 240s or above. In 2011, the mean USMLE Step 1 and 2 scores of matched US Seniors were 243 and 250, respectively. Having an overall strong application is important. Other aspects, such as a unique strength or accomplishment, can also be helpful.

A 2012 publication by Puscas *et al.* [6] has shown that Otolaryngology Program Directors feel that the interview, personal knowledge of the applicant, USMLE scores, LoRs, and medical school grades are the five most important applicant criteria, in that specific order. It is of no surprise that three of the top five criteria (interview, personal knowledge, and LoR) rely on personal interaction with the applicant, either directly or through the author of the LoR.

Insider Tip: Once an applicant receives an interview, he/she is essentially on the same playing field as the other applicants. Be professional, honest, and focused while also letting your personality show through. After a number of interviews, the process can be somewhat grueling, but remember to be engaged and interested.

Extra Insider Tips:
- **Meet the residents if there is a reception, dinner, or other event.** Be polite, honest and, above all, be yourself. Make an effort to speak to a number of residents and faculty members. Some of them are likely on the selection committee.
- **Keep in mind that you could be working side by side with these residents and faculty for years to come.** Imagine yourself working professionally with these individuals. This is what they are likely doing with you. The residents are highly vested in selecting colleagues who will work well with their group.
- **Although not necessary, consider attending a national meeting, such as the Combined Otolaryngologic Sections Meeting (COSM) or the Academy of Otolaryngology Annual Meeting.** These national meetings provide abundant educational experiences. Presenting a poster or oral presentation can be helpful in terms of networking and also strengthening your application.
- **Visit www.otomatch.com during the interview process.** This is an applicant-run website that provides some basic information regarding the interview season. Remember to take the information you read here with a grain of salt, as you do not know who is posting the information and contradictory reports are common.

Chapter 3

References

1. NRMP (2013) *Data Release and Research Committee: Results of the 2013 NRMP Applicant Survey by Preferred Specialty and Applicant Type.* Washington, DC: National Resident Matching Program.
2. NRMP (2013) *Results and Data: 2013 Main Residency Match®.* Washington, DC: National Resident Matching Program.
3. AMGA (2012) *Medical Group Compensation and Financial Survey.* Alexandria, VA: American Medical Group Association.
4. NRMP (2012) *Data Release and Research Committee: Results of the 2012 NRMP Program Director Survey.* Washington, DC: National Resident Matching Program.
5. NRMP (2011) *Charting Outcomes in the Match, 2011.* Washington, DC: National Resident Matching Program.
6. Puscas, L., *et al.* (2012) Qualities of residency applicants: comparison of otolaryngology program criteria with applicant expectations. *Archives of Otolaryngology – Head and Neck Surgery* **138** (1): 10–14.

Pathology

Bonnie Choy, MD and Anthony Chang, MD
Pritzker School of Medicine, University of Chicago, Chicago, IL

Introduction

Pathology is a multifaceted specialty that encompasses every aspect of clinical medicine. Although there are minimal to no direct patient interactions, pathologists are often the physicians who establish the final diagnosis, which tremendously impacts patient management. In addition, approximately 80% of any medical record comprises information that is generated by the Pathology laboratory. The close interactions (intraoperative or formal consultations, tumor boards, and other forums) with clinicians are also rewarding. A successful pathologist must master a large fund of medical knowledge, which is why they are often known as the "doctor's doctor." Anatomic Pathology (AP) encompasses Surgical Pathology, Cytopathology, Dermatopathology, Pediatric Pathology, Neuropathology, and Forensic Pathology. Within Surgical Pathology, there are other subspecialties without additional board certification, including Gastrointestinal, Genitourinary, Breast/Gynecological, Pulmonary, Cardiac, Bone and Soft Tissue, Head and Neck, Transplant, and Medical Renal Pathology. Clinical Pathology (CP), also known as Laboratory Medicine, encompasses Hematopathology, Blood Banking/Transfusion Medicine, Molecular and Genetic Pathology, Microbiology, Clinical Chemistry, Coagulation, and Informatics. However, this traditional boundary between AP and CP is blurring with the introduction of new laboratory and molecular diagnostic tools that span both realms.

The length of residency is 4 years for AP/CP and 3 years for either AP-only or CP-only. The majority of residents pursue AP/CP training, with about 10% in the AP-only and less than 5% in CP-only tracks. No Preliminary or Transitional Year in either Medicine or Surgery is required. Most residents pursue additional fellowship training in either an AP or CP subspecialty. Most fellowships are 1 year in duration, except for the 2-year fellowship in Neuropathology. Recent concerns about a slowing Pathology job market are unwarranted, as the median age of the Pathology workforce is 55 years (third highest among all medical specialties). In fact, a significant shortage of pathologists is anticipated in the near future as the current workforce rapidly approaches retirement age.

Preparation

If you are undecided about a future career in Pathology, complete a Pathology rotation as soon as possible or consider investing a year as a post-sophomore Pathology fellow. This year-long experience will provide insights into the expected duties and responsibilities of a pathologist and make you a better physician, even if you decide to pursue a career in another specialty. If your academic performance during your pre-clinical years or United States Medical Licensing Examination® (USMLE®) scores is below average, or if your medical school is not considered in the top-tier category, completing a post-sophomore Pathology fellowship and obtaining good to excellent evaluations during the process will enhance your application to pathology residency programs. (If you are already in your final year of medical school when you read this, then pursuing a post-sophomore Pathology fellowship might not be the logical next step.) For current offerings of post-sophomore Pathology fellowships, search this term on Google or another internet search engine. Be aware that some programs consider only medical students from their own institution.

Completing one or more Pathology rotations either in the third or fourth year of medical school is essential. This exposure also allows you to establish relationships with Pathology attendings, who may provide letters of recommendation (LoRs) for you. Therefore, if you have a choice, it is better to participate in many Surgical Pathology signout sessions with a few faculty members throughout your rotation, so that they may become better acquainted with you during a short period of time. Set up a meeting with faculty members early in the rotation or even before it starts, to discuss your plan to pursue a career in pathology. If you have an area of interest and are willing to put in the extra effort, ask about suitable research projects. The abstract deadline for the US and Canadian Academy of Pathology (USCAP) Annual Meeting is now in early October, so submitting data from a summer research project is very feasible. The disposition of these submissions is announced in late November, so this can be a nice topic of discussion during your residency interviews if your abstract has been accepted for either a poster or platform presentation. Publication of a manuscript from such a research project would impress any residency Program Director.

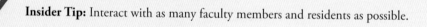

Insider Tip: Interact with as many faculty members and residents as possible.

Obtain information from both faculty members and residents. In particular, the first- and second-year residents have just completed the residency application and interview process, and possess substantial recent knowledge and experience. Also, stay in touch with the recent graduates of your medical school and contact them about their current residency programs.

If you have a definite top choice, consider arranging a Pathology rotation at that institution. This demonstrates initiative and implicitly expresses a strong desire to pursue your residency training there. A good-to-excellent performance will enhance your chances of matching with your top choice and separate you from all of the other applicants on paper.

Most applicants apply for the combined AP/CP pathway. Some residency programs may prefer AP-only or CP-only applicants, as this suggests a greater commitment to an academic career, but this is limited to only a few of the top-tier programs. Programs can differ in their division of AP and CP training. Some programs have either 1- or 2-year blocks of AP or CP rotations, while others have a mixture of AP and CP rotations throughout the year. There are advantages and disadvantages to both schedules, but one system is not necessarily superior to the other.

Applying

In 2013, 583 pathology positions were offered at the PGY-1 level; 45.1% of these positions were filled by US Seniors and 96.4% of the total positions offered were filled. International Medical Graduates (IMGs) filled 35.0% of positions. According to data from the 2012 National Resident Matching Program (NRMP®) *Program Director Survey*, the average program receives 362 applications, interviews 40 candidates and ranks 27 candidates for a class of four residents. In 2011, the mean USMLE Step 1 and 2 scores of matched US Seniors were 226 and 233, respectively [1–5].

Submit your application early. Do not wait for your letters of recommendation to be submitted. Many programs send out invitations for interview even before the Medical Student Performance Evaluation (MSPE) is available on October 1. Therefore, a late submission will decrease your chances to obtain interview invitations.

Ask for your LoRs in August to give your writers plenty of time. Have at least two letters from pathologists. One letter from a non-pathologist is sufficient, as your MSPE will provide enough information about your clinical skills. MD/PhD candidates can have a fourth letter from their PhD mentor.

If you have not received an application status update from a program that is among your top choices by October 15, express your interest in that program by directly emailing the Residency Coordinator and/or Residency Director. This is important if you are interested in a specific geographical area or already have a scheduled interview at another program in the same city or region.

QUICK FACTS

Rank: Less competitive
Median salary: $363 599
Residency years: 4 years (AP/CP) or 3 years (AP-only or CP-only)
Number of residency positions: 583
Number of filled residency positions: 562 (96.4%)
Number filled by US Seniors: 263 (45.1%)
Number of applicants:
  US Seniors: 290
  Total: 949
Ratio of applicants to available positions: 1.6:1
Median number of applications:
  US Seniors: 20
  Independent: 50
Median number of interviews offered:
  US Seniors: 14
  Independent: 8
Median number of programs ranked:
  US Seniors: 9
  Independent: 6
Average resident work hours: 40–50 hours
Average attending work hours: 40 hours
Resident call: Home call
Data based upon [1–3]

Interview

The interview season typically begins in October and lasts until early February for some programs. Do not be surprised if you receive an interview invitation soon after your application submission. There is no advantage to interviewing early and this could become a disadvantage because your impression on a program from a single-day interview may fade with time.

Remember that the interview is also an opportunity for you to learn about the program, faculty, and residents, so that you can determine if the program is a good fit. Be prepared to discuss anything that is included in your application, especially any research or volunteer experience.

Chapter 3

The main factors to consider for residency training include: geography, program size, case load, amount of time you have to preview cases, amount of time spent with faculty versus fellows, number of fellowships offered by the program, cost of living, book fund, and benefits.

> **Insider Tip:** Ensure that there is sufficient preview time for a Surgical Pathology rotation.

It is essential that there is dedicated time for you to preview your Surgical Pathology specimens. If the amount of time that is allotted for this activity is too restricted, that is an undesirable aspect of the program.

Do your homework and research the program as well as the faculty members who may be interviewing you. A great deal of data about the program can be obtained prior to your visit and having this information should allow you to ask more specific questions. This will make your visit more useful, while asking informed questions will impress your interviewers.

Be genuine and polite. The Pathology community is small, so do not offend anyone. Take advantage of the limited time that you will have with the residents on the day of the interview. Ask good questions, as this is the best opportunity to obtain honest answers about the program. In addition, the personalities of the residents will provide the best insight into the character of the residency program. The residents are often as important as the faculty members, as you will be working side by side with them for long periods. Make sure you can see yourself as a part of the program. Do remember that residents evaluate you, so asking questions about vacation or work hours or any inappropriate comments will be noted.

Follow-Up

Write thank you email messages or cards/letters to your interviewers. Stay in touch with the Program Director and/or Program Coordinator (or even residents). If you have a publication, abstract acceptance, or other achievements after your interview, send updates to inform the programs about them.

If you have a top choice, you can voluntarily share this information with that program. In our experience, this usually positively impacts your probability of matching there. If you have a good relationship with a faculty member from your institution, they may be able contact someone at your top choice and reiterate your strong desire to match at that particular program. Do not tell a program that it is your top choice if that is not true.

Second visits may be offered for select applicants. These can be time-consuming and potentially expensive, but this opportunity can provide additional insights about the daily routine at the particular department in a more relaxed atmosphere.

Extra Insider Tips:

- **If you have the rare opportunity to attend the annual meetings of the USCAP or College of American Pathologists as a third-year medical student, attend the fellowship fairs.** Introduce yourself to residency Program Directors, who are often present as representatives of their institutions.
- **If the program offers dinner with the residents the night before your interview day, try your best to attend.** This is a great opportunity to learn about the program from the most important people in that department. Your absence may be perceived in a negative manner, unless you have a great excuse.
- **Be on your best behavior.** The opinions of the residents are highly valued, so be on your best behavior at all times, especially during lunch or at dinner the night before your interview day.
- The **Intersociety Council for Pathology Information** (ICPI; www.pathologytraining.org) offers a complete directory of pathology training programs with a search engine (by institution, state, geographic region).
- The **American Society of Clinical Pathology** (ASCP; www.ascp.org) and the **College of American Pathology** (www.cap.org) provide resources for medical students who are interested in a pathology career.
- **Both the ICPI and the ASCP offer medical student awards.**

References

1. NRMP (2013) *Data Release and Research Committee: Results of the 2013 NRMP Applicant Survey by Preferred Specialty and Applicant Type.* Washington, DC: National Resident Matching Program.
2. NRMP (2013) *Results and Data: 2013 Main Residency Match®.* Washington, DC: National Resident Matching Program.
3. AMGA (2012) *Medical Group Compensation and Financial Survey.* Alexandria, VA: American Medical Group Association.
4. NRMP (2012) *Data Release and Research Committee: Results of the 2012 NRMP Program Director Survey.* Washington, DC: National Resident Matching Program.
5. NRMP (2011) *Charting Outcomes in the Match, 2011.* Washington, DC: National Resident Matching Program.

Chapter 3

Pediatrics

Laura Chen, MD, Amy Downing, MD, and Heather McPhillips, MD, MPH
University of Washington Medical School and Seattle Children's Hospital, Seattle, WA

Introduction

A pediatrician takes care of patients through the spectrum of their childhood and adolescence in a variety of settings, and must partner with parents and caregivers as well as the patient to provide the best pediatric care. Outpatient primary-care pediatricians often focus their practice on prevention of disease, and the diagnosis and treatment of common acute illness. Hospital-based pediatricians (pediatric hospitalists) treat children who are admitted to the hospital. Pediatricians who have received additional specialty training through fellowships typically treat children with complex or chronic diseases, including genetic diseases, developmental disorders, cancer and diseases of the blood, pulmonary conditions such as cystic fibrosis, and disease involving the heart and gastrointestinal tract, to name just a few.

Primary-care pediatricians form long-standing relationships with their patients, seeing them for well-child checks from infancy through teenage years, treating them when they become ill, and guiding patients and their parents through chronic disorders such as diabetes, obesity, asthma, and mental health conditions. Some outpatient pediatricians also follow their patients when they are hospitalized. Pediatricians may attend deliveries and resuscitate babies, truly knowing their patients since the day they were born. Other career options include becoming a hospitalist (working solely as an inpatient provider), teaching medical students and residents in an academic setting, conducting research, or being involved in public health and policy. Many pediatricians go on to pursue subspecialty training in a pediatric fellowship. Your career choices are numerous.

Many medical students choose Pediatrics because they enjoy working with children and families. However, having experience or even comfort interacting with and examining babies and toddlers often takes time. Children are resilient and recover from serious illness quickly, generally with good humor. They are also less likely to have developed health behaviors that cause illness, and many pediatricians enjoy their role in prevention. For example, if a pediatrician can help a child or adolescent avoid smoking until age 18, the chance of that person *ever* smoking is significantly decreased. Likewise, children and families who develop healthy eating habits early in life are less likely to develop obesity and related diseases in adulthood. It takes a certain amount of creativity and flexibility to work with children as they progress through developmental stages. And children are just plain fun.

A residency in General Pediatrics is 3 years. During this time, Pediatrics residents complete monthly rotations including Term Newborn Care, Neonatal Medicine, Hospital Acute Care Wards, Emergency Medicine, Critical Care, Adolescent Medicine, and Developmental Pediatrics, as well as work in a longitudinal outpatient clinic. Due to recent changes in requirements, residency programs in Pediatrics allow for individualized training experiences and may include opportunities to work in depth in Global Child Health, Child Advocacy, and Medical Education in addition to more traditional rotations and electives in subspecialties such as Cardiology, Pulmonary, and Infectious

Diseases. As a Pediatrics resident, you will attend deliveries, resuscitate newborns and critically ill children, and perform procedures such as lumbar punctures, but more importantly, you will learn the medical knowledge and communication skills to become a great pediatrician.

After completing a General Pediatrics residency, about a third continue on to complete a 3-year fellowship. Available fellowships include Adolescent Medicine, Cardiology, Child Abuse Pediatrics, Critical Care Medicine, Developmental-Behavioral Pediatrics, Emergency Medicine, Endocrinology, Gastroenterology, Hematology-Oncology, Infectious Diseases, Neonatology, Nephrology, Pulmonology, and Rheumatology. During residency, you have the opportunity to explore each of these fields as a career during elective months.

> **Insider Tip:** If you would like to go straight through from residency to fellowship, you will apply for some fellowships during your second year and others in your third year of residency.

Preparation

What sets your application apart from others will be demonstrated dedication and leadership in your activities. As most Pediatrics programs highly value advocacy and community service along with more traditional attributes such as scholarly products (presentations and publications), make sure your time spent in the first 2–3 years of medical school includes some meaningful extracurricular activities. Other applicants may have volunteered at a student-run free clinic, but being the Clinic Co-director will set you apart. Many applicants will be members of their school's pediatric interest group, but assuming a leadership position within that group demonstrates your commitment. Longitudinal volunteer experiences also stand out. For example, volunteering for 2 days at a summer camp for children with leukemia does not mean as much as volunteering for 2 years at a smoking cessation clinic. Find an activity you truly enjoy participating in and stick with it. These activities do not have to be related to Pediatrics – commitment and follow through are most important.

Performing well on your third-year core clinical clerkships is important, especially in Pediatrics and Family Medicine. As with all your rotations, be on time, come prepared and ready to learn, read about your patients and their conditions, practice your oral presentations, communicate with patients and families, and be enthusiastic! While many pediatric programs value academic performance highly, grades and United States Medical Licensing Examination® (USMLE®) scores may be somewhat less important than in other specialties if your application is notable for other attributes such as service and leadership.

Throughout your third year of medical school, ask for letters of recommendation (LoRs) from attendings with whom you have worked closely during a rotation. Asking for a letter soon after working with an attending will help them remember specific details so that they can write a strong supporting LoR. Consider providing the faculty member with your draft personal statement and curriculum vitae, as well as reminding your letter writer about a patient or two that you cared for with them as the attending. Including such personal details in a LoR can make your file stand out among the many others that Program Directors read each year. At least one letter should be from the pediatric department, but not all of them must be. Some schools have their Pediatric Department Chair or Clerkship Director write a LoR for their medical students. Find out if this is true at your school and ask for such a letter if this is common practice. The absence of a Chair's or Clerkship Director's letter in your file if everyone else applying in Pediatrics has one will be viewed as a disadvantage by many Program Directors.

 Insider Tip: Consider an away rotation at an institution in which you are highly interested.

Demonstrating a sincere interest in other aspects of medicine also makes your application unique. If you are interested in research, get involved in bench or clinical research during medical school. A publication, poster presentation, or oral presentation is optional, but will help your application stand out. Interests in public policy, global health, or specific pediatric populations, such as adolescents, also make your application memorable.

Insider Tip: If you have any gaps in your training or failing grades, explain them in your application or personal statement.

Applying

In 2013, 2616 Pediatric positions were offered at the PGY-1 level; 70.2% of these positions were filled by US Seniors and 99.6% of the total positions offered were filled. International Medical Graduates (IMGs) filled 18.4% of positions. While often thought of as a female-dominated field, approximately 34% of residents are male. According to data from the 2012 National Resident Matching Program (NRMP®) *Program Director Survey*, the average program receives 965 applications, interviews 160 candidates, and ranks 127 candidates for a class of 13 residents. Programs range widely in size, with some small community programs taking six to eight residents per year and larger university-based programs taking more than 40 [1–5].

QUICK FACTS

Rank: Competitive
Average salary: $220 644
Residency years: 3 years
Number of residency positions: 2616 (categorical)
Number of filled residency positions: 2606 total filled (99.6%)
Number filled by US Seniors: 1837 (70.2%)
Number of applicants:
  US Seniors: 2035
  Total: 3984
Ratio of applicants to available positions: 1.5:1
Median number of applications:
  US Seniors: 22
  Independent: 50
Median number of interviews offered:
  US Seniors: 15
  Independent: 10
Median number of programs ranked:
  US Seniors: 10
  Independent: 7
Average resident work hours: 70–80 hours
Average attending work hours: 40–50 hours
Resident call: In-house
Data based upon [1–3]

Insider Tip: Think about your learning style when looking at the size of a residency. Do you learn best by seeing more patients? If so, consider medium to large residencies. Would you prefer to train at a smaller program?

According to the 2012 NRMP *Program Director Survey*, USMLE scores, LoRs, and the personal statement were the three most important factors in selecting which applicants to interview. Applications are given a thorough review by either a faculty member or resident before a decision is made to invite an applicant for an interview. Reviewers carefully consider step exam scores, clinical grades, the Medical Student Performance Evaluation (MSPE), and research and extracurricular activities. They look for applicants with "the whole package" – no single factor will guarantee you an interview (or rejection). Strict USMLE score cutoffs are rare in pediatrics. In 2011, the mean USMLE Step 1 and 2 scores of matched US Seniors were 221 and 234, respectively.

Insider Tip: Your personal statement can make a big difference. Ask many people, including your pediatric mentors and family members, to read it and provide feedback.

After the interview, Program Directors report that the most important factors for final ranking of applicants were interactions with both faculty and housestaff, interpersonal skills, feedback from current residents, professionalism and ethics, pediatric clerkship grades, and perceived commitment to Pediatrics.

Insider Tip: The interview is crucial for matching into a great Pediatrics residency program, so be prepared to be at your best the entire day! Dress professionally (wear a suit and comfortable shoes) and be courteous to everyone you meet. Be prepared with questions about the program, which will demonstrate your interest.

Most Pediatrics residency interview days are enjoyable and relatively "low-key." You will typically interview with one to three faculty members and some programs will have you interview with a resident as well. You will attend teaching conferences, get a tour of the hospital, and usually have some time to interact with the residents. Most programs offer a social event the night before or after your interview. Try to make as many of these as you can, particularly if you are seriously considering the program. Be aware, however, that although these are not strictly part of your interview, feedback from your interactions during social hours or dinners can be reported to members of admissions committees. Avoid "letting your hair down." Treat these events as a professional event where you should be on your best professional behavior, but also use these events to get a feeling for your overall fit with the residents in the program.

Chapter 3

Extra Insider Tips:

- **Send timely, specific thank you notes after your interview days.** Reference specific parts of your conversation or aspects of the program with which you were impressed. Traditional (paper) thank you cards can go a long way, but email is certainly better than nothing. Avoid typos or casual language, as sometimes these notes end up in your applicant file.

- **Be prepared to talk about anything that you included in your application.** Spend some time thinking about why you chose those activities and how they will make you a better pediatrician. Refresh your memory about the research you did as an undergraduate if you listed it in your application, since interviewers may ask you about it.

- **Take advantage of any opportunities to interact with residents during your interview day.** Attend the social hour if it is offered. Many Pediatrics residencies rely heavily on their housestaff's interactions to rank applicants. In addition, it will help you figure out which program is the best fit for you!

- **Make sure you visit the Medical Student section of American Academy of Pediatrics website** (http://www.aap.org/en-us/about-the-aap/Committees-Councils-Sections/Medical-Students/Pages/default.aspx).

References

1. NRMP (2013) *Data Release and Research Committee: Results of the 2013 NRMP Applicant Survey by Preferred Specialty and Applicant Type.* Washington, DC: National Resident Matching Program.
2. NRMP (2013) *Results and Data: 2013 Main Residency Match®.* Washington, DC: National Resident Matching Program.
3. AMGA (2012) *Medical Group Compensation and Financial Survey.* Alexandria, VA: American Medical Group Association.
4. NRMP (2012) *Data Release and Research Committee: Results of the 2012 NRMP Program Director Survey.* Washington, DC: National Resident Matching Program.
5. NRMP (2011) *Charting Outcomes in the Match, 2011.* Washington, DC: National Resident Matching Program.

Chapter 3

Physical Medicine and Rehabilitation

Rina Bloch, MD
Tufts University School of Medicine, Boston, MA

Introduction

Physical Medicine and Rehabilitation (PMR) is a specialty that focuses on function. The specialty came into existence formally in the 1940s. Its growth was related to both the care of World War II veterans and of survivors of the polio epidemics.

The specialty is quite broad-ranging. Major diagnostic groups of patients that you will treat include, but are not limited to: stroke, spinal cord injury, head trauma, and musculoskeletal problems, such as back, neck, and shoulder pain. Physiatrists (the doctors who specialize in PMR) treat patients with spasticitiy due to a number of central nervous system etiologies – stroke, multiple sclerosis, and cerebral palsy, to name a few. Pediatric physiatrists often see children with cerebral palsy and neuromuscular degenerative diseases. Depending on the practice setting, one may see patients with acute trauma. Physiatrists can have a focus on wound care, sports injuries, or cancer. Thus, the range of patients one is exposed to can be quite broad.

Physiatrists spend their professional lives working closely with multiple other specialists in a team-oriented approach. One generally works in conjunction with physical, occupational, and speech therapists. Depending on the practice setting and diagnostic problems, nursing, social work, neuropsychology, orthotics, and prosthetics may be involved. Thus, this is *not* the specialty for someone who prefers to work alone.

Residency consists of 3 years of training after completion of an internship year (PGY-1). Although most programs begin with PGY-2, there are a few that offer combined internship and residency training. Internships can be done in Internal Medicine, Transitional internships, or General Surgery. As a potential resident, if you elect to do a General Surgery internship, you should be careful to ensure that your Internal Medicine skills are adequate to take care of the variety of medical problems you will encounter on the inpatient wards.

During the 3 years of residency, there is a minimum of 1 year of treating inpatients and 1 year of outpatient experiences. The remaining 12 months are more variable, but will include exposure to electrodiagnostic medicine, particularly learning to perform electromyography (EMG) and nerve conduction velocity (NCV) studies. Residents generally also will spend time on a consultation service. The amount of elective time and the extent of the research requirement vary among programs. A case report or poster presentation may be considered adequate, or the resident may be involved in a long-term project with other researchers.

On call duties will vary from rotation to rotation. When on call, the resident may end up doing weekend rounds on a large number of inpatients, or may in certain rotations be able to take phone call from home with rare trips to the hospital. As physiatrists know more about certain problems, the Emergency Room may ask for consultations on matters such as managing autonomic dysreflexia or caring for indwelling baclofen pumps.

Procedural training during residency generally encompasses peripheral nerve blocks, joint injections, botulinum blocks, and refilling of baclofen pumps. Training in lumbar and cervical epidural steroid injections would commonly be part of a fellowship after residency, though some programs provide more exposure to these procedures. Emerging areas that are not yet part of general residency training or daily practice include the development and implementation of computer-based therapies after stroke, orthotics and prosthetics that are more comparable in function to natural limbs, gait labs, and the development of means to promote regeneration in the neurologic system. Although starting to be used clinically, musculoskeletal ultrasound is in its early stages as a diagnostic modality for rehabilitation medicine. After residency, some residents opt for fellowship training, with common areas being Spinal Cord Injury, Pain, Sports Medicine, Brain Injury, Spine, and Pediatric Rehabilitation.

Following completion of training, some physiatrists work in inpatient rehabilitation hospitals, where they have a designated service of their own patients. Others have an outpatient practice or only do consults. There is usually a mix of at least two components. Consultations may be done in acute care hospitals. Other physiatrists primarily see patients in skilled nursing facilities. Electrodiagnostics may become the primary emphasis of a practice or not be done at all, depending on the physician's individual practice setting.

Lifestyle after residency depends on the practice setting. In an inpatient service, the physiatrist may be the physician responsible for initiating the work up of acute medical problems. The advantage of an inpatient service is that the physiatrist can make a major impact on patients at an important time in their lives. This type of practice also enables the physiatrist to more easily keep abreast of what is going on as the patients work with the various therapies. Following a more defined number of patients in the inpatient rehabilitation hospital setting may provide a more stable income compared to an outpatient clinic.

Preparation

In selecting residents, we want to be certain that the potential resident has a clear idea of the specialty and what the training consists of. As a rotation in PMR is not a portion of the core curriculum, medical students may gain exposure to the field by applying for a competitive summer externship between the first and second years, which can be research or clinically oriented, as well as participate in electives during the third or fourth clinical years. A good understanding of anatomy and neurology (peripheral and central nervous system) is particularly helpful. It is also important to keep up one's skill set in the diagnosis and management of acute medical problems.

Insider Tip: Demonstrate that you have read deeply about the field and ideally have some hands-on experience that is relevant, even if it is as a volunteer outside the medical school offerings.

To assure a good fit between the interests and expectations of the prospective resident and the program, programs want to be certain that a medical student recognizes that PMR is not solely sports medicine or doing injections, but much more encompassing. A medical student who thinks that having physical therapy for a basketball-related knee injury comprises the full range of PMR experiences will be shocked when they actually start training. Part of training includes working with people who have had major injuries or severe disabilities due to illness. The resident needs empathy and an understanding that different cultures, families, and individuals vary in their perceptions of how disabilities are handled day to day.

The resident is expected to be able to handle basic and emergent Internal Medicine problems when on call for an inpatient service at most institutions, the level that would be expected if one successfully completed an internship year. For this reason, programs have concern if the applicant does not have any recent experience with clinical medicine in the United States.

> **Insider Tip:** Most applicants will have had a rotation in PMR before applying. If unable to do a formal rotation before the Electronic Residency Application Service (ERAS®) data must be submitted, be sure to discuss your clinical experiences during your interview.

Applying

In 2013, 103 PMR positions were offered at the PGY-1 level and 294 at the PGY-2 level; 51.3% of these positions were filled by US Seniors and 99.7% of the total positions offered were filled. International Medical Graduates (IMGs) filled 15.5% of PGY-1 positions and 15.9% of PGY-2 positions. According to data from the 2012 National Resident Matching Program (NRMP®) *Program Director Survey*, the average program receives 300 applications, interviews 59 candidates, and ranks 44 candidates for a class of four residents. In 2011, the mean United States Medical Licensing Examination® (USMLE®) scores of matched US Seniors were 214 and 224, respectively [1–5].

Applications are reviewed before candidates are invited for interviews. Ideally one has a letter of reference from a physiatrist. A survey of Program Directors noted that the four most commonly used factors in determining whom to interview were the USMLE Step 1 and 2 scores, as well as the personal statement and letters of recommendation.

QUICK FACTS

Rank: Less competitive
Median salary: $253,750
Residency years: 4 years
Number of residency positions: 397 (103 PGY-1 and 294 PGY-2)
Number of filled residency positions: 396 (99.7%)
Number filled by US Seniors: 204 (51.3%)
Number of applicants for PGY-2:
　US: 242
　Total: 593
Median number of applications:
　US Seniors: 25
　Independent: 30
Median number of interviews offered:
　US Seniors: 16
　Independent: 12
Median number of programs ranked:
　US Seniors: 10
　Independent: 9
Average resident work hours: 40–50 hours
Average attending work hours: 40 hours
Resident call: Home call
Data based upon [1–3]

Chapter 3

> **Insider Tip:** Your ERAS personal statement needs to point out not only why you want to go into PMR, but ideally what you can bring to your training program and the field.

> **Insider Tip:** If there are any unusual circumstances, it is best to address them pre-emptively. If there are gaps in your education, make sure to specify what you were doing.

With its focus on the team, PMR programs look for people who they think will work well as part of a larger group. At the interview, be sure to mention any long-term career goals, though it is perfectly acceptable if you do not yet have a firm sense of this while still a medical student. If there is something special that you bring to the table, mention it. Interviews are a mutual process, to allow the students to decide whether they are good fits for the program and vice versa.

> **Insider Tip:** If there is a get-together the night before the interview, it is an opportunity to find out about daily life in the residency program in a more informal setting.

A career in PMR has many advantages, including the potential to work with all age groups and the opportunity to develop long-term doctor–patient relationships. You will encounter patients and families at a particularly vulnerable time in their lives, dealing with an injury or illness that has caused major changes. The reward of the physiatrist is the fulfillment of effecting a positive change!

> **Extra Insider Tip:**
> - The **American Academy of Physical Medicine and Rehabilitation** (www.aapmr.org) and the **Association of Academic Physiatrists** (www.physiatry.org) are useful sources of information.

References

1. NRMP (2013) *Data Release and Research Committee: Results of the 2013 NRMP Applicant Survey by Preferred Specialty and Applicant Type*. Washington, DC: National Resident Matching Program.
2. NRMP (2013) *Results and Data: 2013 Main Residency Match®*. Washington, DC: National Resident Matching Program.
3. AMGA (2012) *Medical Group Compensation and Financial Survey*. Alexandria, VA: American Medical Group Association.
4. NRMP (2012) *Data Release and Research Committee: Results of the 2012 NRMP Program Director Survey*. Washington, DC: National Resident Matching Program.
5. NRMP (2011) *Charting Outcomes in the Match, 2011*. Washington, DC: National Resident Matching Program.

Chapter 3

Plastic Surgery

Jason S. Barr, MD and Pierre B. Saadeh, MD
New York University School of Medicine, New York, NY

Introduction

Plastic surgeons are specialists who reconstruct, repair, or replace physical defects of form or function, both acquired and congenital. The term "plastic" comes from the Greek word "*plastikos*" which means "to shape or to mold." Interestingly, historical evidence of Plastic Surgery dates at least as far back as 600 BC where Sushruta, an Indian physician, described using forehead skin for reconstruction of nasal defects. This technique is still used today.

Traditionally, Plastic Surgery has been a subspecialty of General Surgery. Until recently, plastic surgeons completed a 5-year General Surgery residency prior to applying for a 2- to 3-year Plastic Surgery fellowship. However, as the techniques of General and Plastic Surgery have diverged with the advent of laparoscopy and non-invasive vascular surgery, integrated Plastic Surgery residencies have taken off [1]. The traditional pathway of combined general and Plastic Surgery residencies still exists, but with each passing year fewer plastic surgeons are trained in this manner and more are accepted directly into Plastic Surgery residency from medical school.

Plastic Surgery is a technically demanding specialty characterized by meticulous attention to detail. It is also distinguished in the scope of surgical innovation. Therefore, Plastic Surgery residency programs search for highly motivated individuals with a proven track record of both surgical and research interest. Plastic Surgery attracts some of the most accomplished medical students.

Contrary to popular belief reflected in the media, plastic surgeons are not simply aesthetic surgeons. Aesthetic surgery is but one subdiscipline within Plastic Surgery. In addition to this area of practice, there are multiple other recognized subdisciplines:

- Burn Surgery
- Craniofacial Surgery
- Hand/Upper Extremity Surgery
- Microsurgery/Reconstructive Surgery
- Pediatric Plastic Surgery
- Reconstructive Transplantation

Plastic Surgery also offers great flexibility in terms of lifestyle opportunities. Some plastic surgeons perform extensive cancer extirpation and reconstruction, with cases that can last upwards of 15–20 hours and schedules that push 70–80 hours per week. Alternatively, some surgeons may have office-based practices with mostly elective cases done on an outpatient basis. Every practice one can imagine on this continuum may be tailored on an individual basis. Some surgeons, mostly at academic medical centers, have practices that focus on basic science, clinical, and/or translational research. Others focus on clinical work and do little research at all. Plastic Surgery is defined by its variability, which facilitates one's ability to mold a career that fits.

Integrated Plastic Surgery residency requires 6 clinical years, with some programs adding a year of dedicated research time in the laboratory. The last 3 clinical years are largely uniform and primarily devoted to Plastic Surgery. The first 3 years, however, are quite variable, with time spent on Plastic Surgery rotations ranging from 3 to 19 months [2]. The majority of the residency will be spent in a hospital setting. A mix of inpatient and outpatient procedures will be seen and performed by each resident. Additionally, residents spend time in ambulatory surgery centers and outpatient clinics/offices. Although not required, many graduates take an additional year-long fellowship in one of the subspecialties listed above, increasing the length of the training process.

Plastic Surgery residency is challenging and residents work long hours. Although programs vary, most residents on Plastic Surgery services can expect to average 60–80 hours per week (the current duty hour limit). In general, Plastic Surgery is a very operative specialty. Unlike General Surgery, in which much care is non-operative, the challenges in Plastic Surgery are largely operative in nature and this is reflected in resident duties. First-year residents spend more time managing patients perioperatively and doing simple procedures. As the years progress, residents spend more time in the Operating Room and less taking care of patients on the floor. The most senior residents, with attending surgeon guidance, are responsible for making most decisions regarding patient care and for planning and performing complex operations.

There is some disparity among Plastic Surgery residencies. Some residency programs afford the bulk of experience in certain subspecialties of strength, although certain minimum requirements for different procedures must be met by all graduating residents. This is secondary to such factors as the practices of the faculty, geographic distribution, and socioeconomics. For example, a resident graduating from one program may have minimal experience under the operating microscope, whereas a resident from another program may be independently capable of harvesting and insetting a microvascular free flap.

Plastic Surgery offers one of the most exciting, fulfilling, and diverse practices of any area in medicine. Plastic surgeons operate on every tissue type, every part of the body from head to toe, and patients from all demographics. The specialty is sometimes said to train "the last true general surgeons." The first kidney transplant was performed by a plastic surgeon, Dr. Joseph Murray, in 1954. Now, with the advent of extremity and facial transplantation, Plastic Surgery is once again establishing new frontiers. One can expect a life of variety in a field that is always changing and pushing innovation.

Insider Tip: Do not immediately rule out a career in Plastic Surgery because you are afraid that it is too difficult to get into the field. The range of Plastic Surgery residents is varied and the diligent can ultimately succeed.

Chapter 3

Preparation

Pre-Clinical Years

A frequent rumor is that "nobody cares about grades" or "P = MD" during the pre-clinical years. While it is true that a passing grade will get you through medical school, it will not get you into the most competitive specialties. Strive to always know as much as possible on every subject and score at the top on every exam. Additionally, pre-clinical grades are often factored into Alpha Omega Alpha Honor Society decisions during the third/fourth year. If offered at your school, Alpha Omega Alpha can be helpful in getting into Plastic Surgery and according to a 2008 questionnaire of Program Directors is the most important objective criterion used in selecting residents [3]. According to the National Resident Matching Program (NRMP®), almost 50% of successfully matched applicants in Plastic Surgery are members of this honor society.

Although "free time" is not in abundance in medical school, smart allocation of this time can include a focus on research. Not only will this help you build an important skill set, but you will foster early relationships with mentors who can help you develop your interest and ultimately your application. It is often stated that it is "absolutely necessary" to take a year or two off from medical school for research in order to get into Plastic Surgery. This is *not* true. In fact, by using some free time during your first 2 years of medical school, you can get involved in Plastic Surgery research and set yourself up for a residency position without committing to extra time for research.

> **Insider Tip:** Try to meet and speak with an individual with an established research track record at the beginning of medical school and express your interest. This includes faculty or a resident generally beyond PGY-2. The residency Program Director can often help with this. Work hard on a research project with this individual and you will find that for the rest of medical school you have a reliable source of research opportunities flowing your way!

Clinical Years

During your clinical years, give your all in every rotation. Try to "honor" as many of the core clerkships as possible. It is a strong show of ability to "honor" not only Surgery and Plastic Surgery, but Medicine, Pediatrics, Obstetrics and Gynecology, and other subjects, and this is scrutinized by many Program Directors. During residency, you will not always be on a rotation that you like. In this scenario, the program still needs to know that you will give 110% for the patients. This demonstrates your intellectual fortitude and your ability to work well with a variety of people. So buckle down and try to do well in all core clerkships.

> **Insider Tip:** The world of medicine is small and the Plastic Surgery match is difficult even for the ideal candidate. Keep your attitude up and your head down and good things will come your way.

Your performance on Plastic Surgery subinternships is an important part of your application for three reasons: (1) if you perform well, the places you rotate are the places where you are most likely to match [4], (2) excellent work on a subinternship can translate into a letter of recommendation that is strong and helps you at other places, and (3) your "fit" with a program is likely to be ascertained. In a 2008 study by Janis *et al.* [5], the most important factors considered by Plastic Surgery Program Directors when selecting residents were letters of recommendation (LoRs) and performance on subinternship. So work hard and have fun!

> **Insider Tip:** In many programs, your greatest exposure will be to the resident teams. Feedback from the residents will be critical to a program's assessment of your performance and, probably more importantly, your "fit" with a program.

The age-old adage in surgery of "the three A's" is as appropriate as any: affable, available, and able. On your rotations, be friendly and helpful. People enjoy working with positive people. Be the first one at the hospital in the morning and the last to leave. Anticipate the needs of your team without being annoying about it. We notice when a student puts his/her head down and works hard.

> **Insider Tip:** Emulate the behavior of your predecessors who have successfully navigated their way into Plastic Surgery. Ask them questions and reproduce the formula that has worked in the past. While there are a great variety of people with differing interests in Plastic Surgery, there is a set of principles and ideals that applies to most.

United States Medical Licensing Examination® (USMLE®) Examinations

There is no doubt that high USMLE scores are very important to be successful in the Plastic Surgery match [6–8]. In the 2011 NRMP *Charting Outcomes in the Match*, the average USMLE Step 1 score for successfully matched US Seniors was 249. Furthermore, there is a linear increase in probability of a successful match as USMLE Step 1 score increases. There is no secret to doing well on this exam. Like all things, hard work pays off.

USMLE Step 2 is a less important part of the equation. In the 2011 NRMP *Charting Outcomes in the Match*, the majority of applicants had not taken USMLE Step 2 at the time of the match. If you score very high on USMLE Step 1, it can be to your disadvantage to take

Step 2 prior to the Match. On the other hand, if you have high USMLE Step 1 and 2 scores, your consistency and your implied confidence in your knowledge base will be noticed. Finally, if you have a mediocre USMLE Step 1 score, knocking Step 2 out of the park may help you. It is important to note that many (but not all) programs use a cutoff USMLE Step 1 score to help filter the many applications they receive. For example, our institution receives over 200–250 applications each year for approximately 22–24 interview spots and three positions. Although we do not have an absolute "cutoff" number, we are not likely to consider applicants with USMLE scores below 220.

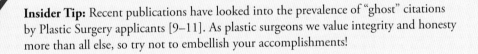

> **Insider Tip:** The more you read and study, the higher your USMLE scores will be!

Research Experience

According to the 2011 NRMP *Charting Outcomes in the Match*, the mean number of research experiences for successfully matched US Seniors was 3.8 (3.7 for unsuccessful applicants). Further, the mean number of abstracts, publications, and presentations was 8.7 (6.1 for unsuccessful applicants). Do not let these numbers intimidate you! For every accepted applicant who has 15 publications, there is another who has only one. It is not the number that is important, so much as the quality and your ability to explain what you did for a research project during an interview.

> **Insider Tip:** Recent publications have looked into the prevalence of "ghost" citations by Plastic Surgery applicants [9–11]. As plastic surgeons we value integrity and honesty more than all else, so try not to embellish your accomplishments!

LoRs

These are one of the most important parts of your application [12]. When applying to Plastic Surgery, there are a few guidelines to follow when considering who ought to write your letters of recommendation. First, you are allowed up to four letters and three are required. In general, letters from plastic surgeons carry more weight than those from non-plastic surgeons. Make sure your letter writer knows you well and can support your application. It is also helpful, but not required, if the person writing one of the letters is well-known in the field of academic Plastic Surgery.

> **Insider Tip:** There is a "standard" LoR that Program Directors must use and that other letter writers are encouraged to use. This letter is relatively objective, so make sure you will get one that strengthens your application (*ask!*). If it will not at least strengthen your application, you are doing yourself a significant disservice.

Chapter 3

Applying

When applying to a specialty as competitive as Plastic Surgery, it is important to have a viable "backup plan." The match can be capricious, and highly qualified individuals may not match in any particular year. Moreover, even if you are the strongest applicant in the pool, you *will* be asked about your backup plan in your interviews. It does not really matter what your backup plan is, so long as you have one. It can range from applying to General Surgery or another specialty in addition to Plastic Surgery, or to taking 1 or 2 years off for research. Plastic surgeons make their living by having backup plans in place in case a given procedure fails to adequately address a given clinical problem, so you must have one as well.

QUICK FACTS

Rank: Highly competitive
Median salary: $409 772
Residency years: 6–7 years (Integrated Residency)
Number of residency positions: 127 (116 PGY1 and 11 PGY2)
Number of filled residency positions: 126 (99.2%)
Number filled by US Seniors: 121 (95.3%)
Number of applicants:
  US Seniors: 179
  Total: 203
Median number of applications:
  US Seniors: 53
  Independent: 55
Median number of interviews offered:
  US Seniors: 18
  Independent: 3
Median number of programs ranked:
  US Seniors: 12
  Independent: 4
Average resident work hours: 60–80 hours
Average attending work hours: 60 hours
Resident call: In-house
Data based on [14–16]

 Insider Tip: When it comes to dual application in another specialty, even though a recent study found that the number of applicants dual applying is decreasing [13], you must have a backup plan so you do not find yourself "scrambling" into an undesirable residency spot through the Supplemental Offer and Acceptance Program (SOAP®).

According to the NRMP data, in 2013, 127 positions were offered at the PGY-1 (116) and PGY-2 (11) levels. Of these, 121 were filled by US Seniors (95.3%) and six by independent applicants [14–18].

Given the small size of the field of Plastic Surgery, as well as its competitive nature, the conventional wisdom is to apply to as many programs as you can afford. ERAS charges applicants based on the number of residencies applied to under the same specialty. Although Plastic Surgery leadership recognizes the cost burden in this process, a viable less-expensive alternative has not been identified.

 Insider Tip: Although expensive, you only get one opportunity to apply to integrated Plastic Surgery residency as a US Senior, so make it count!

Interviews

According to the NRMP 2012 *Program Director Survey*, the interview performance is the most important factor in deciding how highly to rank an applicant. Try your best to relax and be yourself. There are a number of questions you *must* have an answer to:

- Tell me about yourself.
- Why Plastic Surgery?
- There are lots of good applicants here, what makes you unique?
- Why our program?
- What if you do not match?
- What did you do for this research project?

Remember, once you get to the interview, it is a much more even playing field. The interviewers want to know the real you. Moreover, they want to know if the real you will likely mesh well in their residency program. When you walk into the interview, enter with a smile and your head held high. Most interviewers will tell you that within 3–4 minutes of meeting an interviewee, he/she knows how highly to rank that person based on interview skills. Exude confidence and be friendly.

Unfortunately, matching in Plastic Surgery is a numbers game. This means that you ought to attend as many interviews as you possibly can handle/afford. Multiple published studies in addition to the NRMP data demonstrate that the more interviews an applicant attends, the higher the match rate.

As a final note, during interviews you are allowed to express your level of interest in the program. Similarly, your interviewers can express interest in you. However, communication regarding rank intentions between applicants and programs is not allowed after the interview day. So your interest must be made clear on interview day. Then relax and consider your rank list order!

 Insider Tip: Refrain from saying anything negative about anyone or anything. Remember, positivity is essential!

References

1. Luce, E. A. (1995) Integrated training in plastic surgery: concept, implementation, benefits, and liabilities. *Plastic and Reconstructive Surgery* **95** (1): 119–123.
2. Schneider, L. F., *et al.* (2013) A nationwide curriculum analysis of integrated plastic surgery training: is training standardized? *Plastic and Reconstructive Surgery* **132** (6): 1054e–1062e.
3. LaGrasso, J. R., *et al.* (2008) Selection criteria for the integrated model of plastic surgery residency. *Plastic and Reconstructive Surgery* **121** (3): 121e–125e.
4. Wood, J. S. and David, L. R. (2010) Outcome analysis of factors impacting the plastic surgery match. *Annals of Plastic Surgery* **64** (6): 770–774.
5. Janis, J. E. and Hatef, D. A. (2008) Resident selection protocols in plastic surgery: a national survey of plastic surgery Program Directors. *Plastic and Reconstructive Surgery* **122** (6): 1929–1939; discussion 1940–1921.

Chapter 3

6. Rinard, J. R. and Mahabir, R. C. (2010) Successfully matching into surgical specialties: an analysis of national resident matching program data. *Journal of Graduate Medical Education* **2** (3): 316–321.

7. Claiborne, J. R., *et al.* (2013) The plastic surgery match: predicting success and improving the process. *Annals of Plastic Surgery* **70** (6): 698–703.

8. Rogers, C. R., *et al.* (2009) Integrated plastic surgery residency applicant survey: characteristics of successful applicants and feedback about the interview process. *Plastic and Reconstructive Surgery* **123** (5): 1607–1617.

9. Phillips, J. P., *et al.* (2012) Misrepresentation of scholarly works by integrated plastic surgery applicants. *Plastic and Reconstructive Surgery* **130** (3): 731–735.

10. Larson, J. D., *et al.* (2010) The presence of "ghost" citations in an applicant pool of an integrated plastic surgery residency program. *Plastic and Reconstructive Surgery* **126** (4): 1390–1394.

11. Adetayo, O. A. (2011) The presence of "ghost" citations in an applicant pool of an integrated plastic surgery residency program. *Plastic and Reconstructive Surgery* **127** (5): 2137–2138; author reply 2138.

12. Nguyen, A. T. and Janis, J. E. (2012) Resident selection protocols in plastic surgery: a national survey of plastic surgery independent Program Directors. *Plastic and Reconstructive Surgery* **130** (2): 459–469.

13. Super, N., *et al.* (2013) Recent trends in applicants and the matching process for the integrated plastic surgery match. *Annals of Plastic Surgery* **71** (4): 406–409.

14. NRMP (2013) *Data Release and Research Committee: Results of the 2013 NRMP Applicant Survey by Preferred Specialty and Applicant Type.* Washington, DC: National Resident Matching Program.

15. NRMP (2013) *Results and Data: 2013 Main Residency Match®.* Washington, DC: National Resident Matching Program.

16. AMGA (2012) *Medical Group Compensation and Financial Survey.* Alexandria, VA: American Medical Group Association.

17. NRMP (2012) *Results and Data: 2012 Main Residency Match®.* Washington, DC: National Resident Matching Program.

18. NRMP (2011) *Charting Outcomes in the Match, 2011.* Washington, DC: National Resident Matching Program.

Chapter 3

Psychiatry

Jennifer L. Kurth, DO
Northwestern University Feinberg School of Medicine, Chicago, IL

Introduction

Psychiatry is a specialty area of medicine focused on the diagnosis and treatment of mental, addictive, and emotional disorders. Psychiatrists incorporate biological, psychological, and sociocultural components into the assessment and treatment of mental illness. Being physicians, psychiatrists are qualified to order diagnostic laboratory tests, perform procedures such as electroconvulsive therapy (ECT) and transcranial magnetic stimulation, and prescribe medications as indicated to treat psychiatric illnesses. In addition, psychiatrists provide psychotherapy treatments, and are prepared to support individuals dealing with life stresses and crises. Clinically, psychiatrists can work in a variety of settings including community- and academic-based hospitals, residential treatment centers, community mental health centers, college campus mental health centers, outpatient facilities, detention centers, and nursing homes, as well as in private practice. Owing to this versatility, psychiatrists can engage in both short- and long-term care for patients. Psychiatrists can also choose to pursue careers in research, forensics, mental health administration in public and private settings, and academics.

It is a very exciting time to train in Psychiatry. As a field, we are continually gaining a greater understanding of brain functioning and the etiologic role of genetics, epigenetics, and environmental factors in the onset of psychiatric illness. Furthermore, the ongoing development of effective therapy modalities, medications, and procedures provides many more treatment options. Being a psychiatrist is much like being a detective, and one must be curious and constantly asking questions and reading between the lines to understand the development and role of psychiatric symptoms in the patient's life. Psychiatrists utilize this level of detail to synthesize an assessment and case formulation for the patient's presenting condition. Psychiatrists use the *Diagnostic and Statistical Manual of Mental Disorders* [1] to make diagnoses. Diagnosis is often a challenging and complex process, though this is often what drives people into the field. Psychiatrists thrive on these challenges and there is no such thing as clinical monotony or boredom in our field.

Residency training is 4 years long (unless one transfers into a Child and Adolescent Psychiatry fellowship after 3 years of adult training), and provides clinical experiences, supervision, and formal didactics covering all areas of Psychiatry. Although most residents enter Psychiatry programs at the postgraduate year PGY-1 level, it is possible to enter a program at the PGY-2 level, generally following an intern or Transitional Year in Medicine, Family Practice or Pediatrics.

PGY-1 in Psychiatry consists of 4 months of a primary-care experience, 2 months of Neurology, and 6 months of Psychiatry. The "primary-care experience" can include Family Medicine, Internal Medicine, and/or Pediatrics. One month of the primary-care experience can be done in Emergency Medicine, Intensive Care, or Medical Consult Patient Care. Programs vary widely in how PGY-2 to PGY-4 are scheduled and the types of clinical experiences offered. Some programs are "front-loaded" to get most of the call and intensive service rotations completed early to allow for more flexible time in PGY-3 and PGY-4. Other programs have intensive service rotations throughout the training experience, while some meet subspecialty clinical requirements by using outpatient versus inpatient experiences. It is required that all programs offer a 12-month longitudinal, continuous outpatient experience, though some programs allow residents to start longitudinal treatment with patients as early as PGY-2. Some programs have many faculty available for supervision, while others rely on a few core faculty to supervise multiple experiences. Some programs have been unstable in the past with many faculty and residents leaving, while others have little turnover. Some programs have been known to focus more on Biological or Psychodynamic Psychiatry, rather than a balance of the two.

All of the above factors can create vastly different learning experiences. Programs vary greatly with regards to the call schedule, though applicants should be cautioned against utilizing this as a primary tool for evaluating a program. In the long run, the quality of training is really a product of the breadth and depth of the clinical experience combined with good supervision and teaching.

> **Insider Tip:** It is important to investigate and differentiate the clinical experiences in each program and the rotations scheduled in PGY-2 to PGY-4 to determine the "best fit" for your education and learning.

Many psychiatrists continue training beyond the initial 3–4 years. After PGY-3, resident can "fast track" into a Child and Adolescent Psychiatry fellowship program. If you are interested in "fast-tracking" after PGY-3 to a Child Psychiatry fellowship, it is important to know that potential programs can assure that you meet all of your Adult Psychiatry requirements by the end of PGY-3. After PGY-4, residents can enter fellowship programs in the areas of Child and Adolescent Psychiatry, Geriatric Psychiatry, Forensic Psychiatry, Addictions Psychiatry, Psychosomatic Medicine, and Pain. There are many "non-Accreditation Council for Graduate Medical Education (ACGME)"-accredited fellowships in areas of Women's Psychiatry and School Mental Health for residents interested in these special clinical areas.

Given that there is significant variation in Psychiatry training programs, it is very important for applicants to decide what factors are most important to them. Applicants should seek guidance from a Psychiatry Training Director, mentor, or career advisor in Psychiatry at their school. It may be helpful for applicants to develop a list of potential programs and then start to differentiate them. Important sources of information include FREIDA Online® (Fellowship and Residency Electronic Interactive Database), which is an online American Medical Association (AMA) database of accredited Graduate Medical Education (GME) programs and their websites. Recent graduates from your medical school who are Psychiatry residents can provide a great deal of information as well. It can be helpful to network with other applicants who have visited programs, as well as with attending physicians who came from other programs. Sitting down again with a Psychiatry Advisor can help the applicant to determine whether their rank list is compatible with their goals and the likelihood of matching.

> ✓ **Insider Tip:** Having a mentor can help with deciding on a "good fit" for training.

Preparation

Psychiatry is a required clerkship during the third year of medical school and usually when students initially develop an interest in the field. To get even more experience, it is a good idea for fourth-year students to consider doing a subinternship rotation or elective. Students may choose to do an externship at an outside potential program of interest to gain more experience, as well as get a closer look at their residency program. This can be a great way to impress a program with your hard work and talent, thus becoming a more competitive candidate for residency.

There are opportunities in medical school to become involved in student interest groups, such as "PsychSIGN" (see website below) as well as student members of such national organizations as the American Psychiatric Association (APA). Free for medical students, APA membership offers access to *The American Journal of Psychiatry* and *Psychiatric News*, free registration to the Annual Meeting, and discounts on psychiatric textbooks. On the APA website, there also are listings of externships and travel awards available for medical students. Medical students who are interested in Child and Adolescent Psychiatry can join the American Academy of Child and Adolescent Psychiatry (AACAP) without cost, as well as have free access to periodicals and registration to the AACAP Annual Meeting.

Students can gain insights into the profession by getting involved in any number of extracurricular activities. This can include doing community outreach, volunteering, providing community service, leadership, teaching, and life experiences. Students may also have opportunities to get involved in research, which is eye catching to Program Directors. It is also highly valuable to present a poster at a national conference, where an applicant can network and demonstrate academic interests and activity.

> ✓ **Insider Tip:** Get involved in extracurricular activities. Academic, community, and volunteer experiences will make your application stand out.

It is a good idea to find faculty mentors at either your own program or an outside psychiatric program of interest. Mentors can help facilitate opportunities for further learning, research, and training. They also can provide more personalized letters of recommendation the longer they know and work with applicants, which is attractive to Program Directors, as well as help an applicant review and consider programs that will provide a good fit for training.

Chapter 3

Applying

A total of 681 US Seniors "matched" into Psychiatry residencies at the PGY1 level (only 2 PGY2 spots were available) in the 2013 National Resident Matching Program (NRMP®). This was an increase from 616 in 2012, reflecting a rise from 3.9 to 4.2% of Seniors selecting careers in Psychiatry. The uptick in graduates entering the profession is good news for Psychiatry, reversing a trend of several years in which the numbers were dropping [2–9].

Starting with the 2013 Match, there is now an "All In Policy" stating that all PGY-1 positions and PGY-2 positions in specialties that can begin at either at the PGY-1 or PGY-2 level must be placed in the Main Residency Match®. In the past, US allopathic Seniors could only obtain a position through the Match, whereas "independent applicants" (non-US allopathic Seniors) could sign contracts outside of the Match. The "All In Policy" was created to level the playing field, so that programs now must place all positions in the Match or none at all.

QUICK FACTS

Rank: Less competitive
Average salary: $217 194
Residency years: 4 years (including Preliminary)
Number of categorical residency positions: 1360 (PGY1)
Number of filled residency positions: 1330 (97.8%)
Number filled by US Seniors: 681 (50.1%)
Number of applicants:
  US Seniors: 749
  Total: 2348
Ratio of applicants to available residency positions: 1.7:1
Median number of applications:
  US Seniors: 20
  Independent: 45
Median number of interviews offered:
  US Seniors: 14
  Independent: 8
Median number of programs ranked:
  US Seniors: 9
  Independent: 6
Average resident work hours: 40–50 hours
Average attending work hours: 40 hours
Resident call: In-house
Data based on [2–4]

The "All In Policy" resulted in more slots offered in the match. In Psychiatry, 1360 positions were offered (compared with 1118 in 2012) and 1330 (97.8%) were filled; 50.1% of these positions were filled by US Seniors, and 97.8% of the total positions offered were filled. International Medical Graduates (IMGs) filled 29.8% of the total positions. According to data from the 2012 NRMP *Program Director Survey*, the average program receives 664 applications, interviews 68 candidates, and ranks 50 candidates for a class of six residents.

Psychiatry residency programs use Electronic Residency Application Service (ERAS®) and the NRMP website to view applications and submit rank lists like most other programs. Most selection committees will want to know about gaps in an applicant's curriculum vitae (CV) or leaves of absences/gaps in time during medical school. Be prepared to discuss any gaps during the interview. Many students utilize the personal statement for explaining any gaps or deficiencies in their application, though it is also perfectly acceptable to discuss this in person with the training director. A strong applicant generally has demonstrated interest in Psychiatry as manifested by community involvement, volunteering, humanistic projects, and research. Even hobbies that make you unique are good to mention to demonstrate your personal roundedness.

Personal statements are very important in the application process for Psychiatry residency and allow Program Directors to have a closer look at you as an applicant. It is a great

Chapter 3

opportunity to introduce yourself in writing to the Program Director and discuss your interests in Psychiatry. Many choose to talk about an experience that broadened their interest in, or understanding of, Psychiatry. It is great to talk about what got you interested in Psychiatry, your career goals and personal strengths. It is not a venue to discuss political or controversial topics, or to demonstrate skill in haiku or poetry. Make sure that a mentor or colleague reads and edits your personal statement. Your personal statement should accurately reflect you, in both structure and content, and make you shine.

United States Medical Licensing Examination® (USMLE®) scores are required for acceptance to a program. While high scores are impressive, most Psychiatry Program Directors do not weigh them heavily for interview selection and applicant ranking. In 2011, the mean USMLE scores of matched US Seniors were 214 and 225, respectively.

> **Insider Tip:** Psychiatry programs like to see applicants who are strong academically, but who also have well-written personal statements and demonstrate character and humanistic interest.

For Psychiatry training programs, the interview is the most important part of the application process. Psychiatrists spend their entire day communicating and interacting with patients, families, treatment teams, and colleagues. It is important for patients to feel comfortable communicating with their psychiatrists and communication problems can be detrimental to patient care. Program Directors want to have residents who are friendly, calm, cooperative, flexible, and good listeners who are eager to learn. Having good interpersonal and communication skills is essential in assessing and diagnosing patients and engaging them in treatment. Program Directors want to see how you can talk and relate to others. Just be yourself!

> **Insider Tip:** The interview and everything associated with it is extremely important!

> **Extra Insider Tips:**
> - **Do your research on the program prior to the interview.** It is so impressive when an applicant comes to interview and it is obvious that they have done their homework on our program. It also makes for a more fruitful interview day, as applicants can have more specific questions prepared and gather more information about areas of interest. Also, if you have a specific area of interest, you can contact the program ahead of time to request possibly meeting with a faculty member in that field during your interview day.
> - **Be prepared to ask a lot of questions.** The most common negative comment I get from faculty interviewers is "I can't believe the applicant did not have any questions!"

Chapter 3

The interview day can be a great opportunity to learn more about both the program and psychiatry in general. Some faculty interviewers may not be as familiar with the nuts and bolts of the training program, but all faculty generally are seeing patients and/or doing research. Talking with them about their special interests, patient care population, or research projects is a great way to learn more about the program and psychiatry in general, while at the same time demonstrating your interest in the program. There is a web link below from the APA website that has a lot of sample questions.

- **Professionalism is key.** This may seem obvious, but you would be surprised how often applicants struggle with professionalism on the interview day. Many programs are chagrined after seeing a candidate who is great on paper present so negatively on interview day. Here are some tips. Even if the program where you are interviewing is at the bottom of your rank list, treat them as if they are on top. If a program senses disinterest or a condescending attitude from the applicant, it is a real turn-off. Interactions with the residents during a lunch and/or dinner are taken into consideration during the selection process. This is important to remember, since it is not like a true "interview session."

Important Websites

- **PsychSIGN:** psychsign.drupalgardens.com
- **American Psychiatric Association:** www.psych.org
- **Sample questions for interview day**: http://www.psych.org/medical-students/applying-for-psychiatry-residency
- **American Academy of Child and Adolescent Psychiatry:** www.aacap.org
- **FREIDA Online:** https://www.ama-assn.org/go/freida

References

1. APA (2013) *Diagnostic and Statistical Manual of Mental Disorders*, 5th edn. Arlington, VA: American Psychiatric Association.
2. NRMP (2013) *Results and Data: 2013 Main Residency Match®*. Washington, DC: National Resident Matching Program.
3. NRMP (2013) *Data Release and Research Committee: Results of the 2013 NRMP Applicant Survey by Preferred Specialty and Applicant Type*. Washington, DC: National Resident Matching Program.
4. AMGA (2012) *Medical Group Compensation and Financial Survey*. Alexandria, VA: American Medical Group Association.
5. NRMP (2012) *Data Release and Research Committee: Results of the 2012 NRMP Program Director Survey*. Washington, DC: National Resident Matching Program.
6. NRMP (2011) *Charting Outcomes in the Match, 2011*. Washington, DC: National Resident Matching Program.
7. Bak, M. K., *et al.* (2006) Applying to psychiatry residency programs. *Academic Psychiatry* **30**: 239–247.
8. Haviland, M. G., *et al.* (2009) Faculty salaries in psychiatry and all clinical science departments, 1980–2006. *Academic Psychiatry* **33**: 157–159.
9. Moran, M. (2013) More graduates choose psychiatry in 2013 match. *Psychiatric News – Professional News*, April 19.

Radiology

Jim S. Wu[a], MD and Suzanne Long[b], MD
[a]Beth Israel Deaconess Medical Center, Harvard Medical School, Boston, MA
[b]Thomas Jefferson University Hospital, Jefferson Medical College, Philadelphia, PA

Introduction

Radiology utilizes a variety of diagnostic and image-guided therapeutic procedures across multiple modalities (ultrasound, computed tomography, magnetic resonance, and fluoroscopy) to participate in patient care from a more removed, consultant standpoint. However, while pursuing a career in Radiology means sacrificing some one-on-one patient interaction, it affords you the opportunity to influence the care of a much greater number of patients with a vast array of pathologies.

Successful radiologists have a keen ability to translate two-dimensional images into three-dimensional structures (organic chemistry may have been useful after all). They have an eye for pattern recognition and attention to detail, and especially excel in self-directed learning. Radiologists have to master a wide range of differential diagnoses across a multitude of specialties, an accomplishment that requires lifelong study. Therefore, Radiology residency programs are looking for the student who has demonstrated academic ability and focus through excellent grades, high board scores, and completed research projects. In addition to the high level of accomplishment expected in an applicant, the specialty is competitive due to the attractiveness of perceived salary and lifestyle.

Radiology is one of the few fields that demonstrate a tremendous difference between academic and private practice workloads and salary, a difference which greatly skews salary reports. The pay scale is also different within private practice groups themselves, with partners often earning double the salary of their academic counterparts. However, before weighing this monetary benefit too heavily in deciding your chosen specialty, be aware that radiologists have been deeply affected by insurance reimbursement restructuring and many of the high salaries of yesteryear will be long gone by the time you finish training. To compensate for these reimbursement cuts, radiologists have had to increase the volume of studies read. An academic radiologist at our academic institution will typically read between 40–60 cross-sectional studies per day, while private practice counterparts often read well above 100. To achieve these numbers, a private practice radiologist often must work very late into the evening on a daily basis.

Residency is 5 years long, consisting of a Preliminary or Transitional Year in Medicine or Surgery and 4 years of Diagnostic Radiology training, which is primarily hospital-based. There is a substantial amount of exposure to procedures throughout residency training, ranging from mammography-guided biopsies to complex angiographic interventions. Therefore, solid hand–eye coordination is a bonus during your residency years. Nevertheless, there are several subspecialties that are based purely on image interpretation. After finishing residency, nearly all go on to perform a 1-year subspecialty fellowship in such areas as Body Imaging,

Chest and Cardiac Radiology, Interventional Radiology (IR), Mammography, Musculoskeletal Imaging, Neuroradiology Imaging and Intervention (2 Years), Nuclear Medicine, or Pediatrics.

The training requirements for IR subspecialization deserve special attention, as they have recently undergone major changes. Currently, residents can pursue IR training via the traditional pathway described above or the lesser-known DIRECT pathway (Diagnostic and Interventional Radiology Enhanced Clinical Training). The DIRECT program requires 2 years of Preliminary clinical training rather than 1 year and can be entered immediately after graduation from medical school or as a PGY-3, for a total of 6 postgraduate training years. In 2012, however, the American Board of Medical Specialties (ABMS) approved the Interventional Radiology/Diagnostic Radiology (IR/DR) Certificate recognizing IR as a "unique medical specialty addressing the diagnosis and treatment of diseases through expertise in diagnostic imaging, image-guided minimally invasive procedures, and the evaluation and clinical management of patients with conditions amenable to these methods" [1]. The plan is replace the current VIR ("Vascular IR") certificate obtained after a 1-year IR fellowship with a distinct IR *residency* which will consist of 3 years of DR and 2 years of IR. The latter will include additional training requirements such as critical care medicine, periprocedural care, and increased IR exposure. The plan is to begin implementing this pathway by July 2015. Each individual residency program will have to decide whether to participate in this new training regimen, with the understanding that the older model will be phased out over the next 5 years. When applying to Radiology residencies, be sure to inquire if and how the program will respond to these new requirements. This is true even if you plan on pursuing DR, as losing a classmate to IR training after completing the third year may affect your call schedule.

A typical hospital-based workday for the DR resident usually spans 8–5 p.m., with 1 hour (or more) per day devoted to resident conferences. However, after leaving the hospital at 5 p.m., you will likely have to continue working from home, editing reports and studying. The number of hours each day required for these activities will depend on your level of efficiency and study habits. DR residents have no call during the first year of residency (PGY-2) – a nice change after an arduous intern year. Call begins during the second year of radiology training and many programs now have 24-hour in-house attending coverage. The exact duties of the overnight attending versus the overnight resident will differ from institution to institution, but generally the attending will supervise the overnight resident in some capacity. For instance, during overnight call, residents are expected to provide preliminary interpretations on imaging studies. The overnight attending may review all of the preliminary reports shortly after they are generated or may only provide timely review of the more difficult cases at the request of the resident, reserving the bulk of the review for the end of the call shift. The logistics are quite variable. This relatively new trend of in-house overnight attending coverage has positive and negative effects on your training: while ideally it improves report turnaround time and reduces the chance of suboptimal or delayed management due to an incorrect preliminary resident report, it does detract from a resident's opportunity for autonomy and simulation of the post-training experience.

Radiology is one of the more family-friendly residencies. The rotation schedule is more flexible than higher-intensity specialties. A significant portion of work and study is spent at home, making Radiology generally more conducive to family obligations.

Preparation

High Pass or Honors on clinical rotations, especially Medicine, Surgery, and Radiology, is extremely important. Demonstrating commitment to the specialty through research during medical school is also helpful. A number of medical student radiology awards are available through such organizations as the Association of University Radiologists (AUR) and the Radiologic Society of North America (RSNA). Away rotations at highly competitive programs may be helpful if you are a solid candidate from a medical school that is not highly ranked. At our institution, we look favorably on outside applicants who have rotated through our department, and demonstrated medical knowledge and initiative that has impressed both residents and attendings.

Applying

In 2013, 1143 diagnostic radiology positions were offered at the PGY-1 (combined with a Preliminary Year) and PGY-2 levels; 72.2% of these positions were filled by US medical seniors and 94.3% of the total positions offered were filled. International Medical Graduates (IMGs) filled 13.4% of PGY-1 radiology positions and 10.4% of PGY-2 positions. According to data from the 2012 National Resident Matching Program (NRMP®) *Program Director Survey*, the average program receives 458 applications, interviews 77 candidates, and ranks 64 candidates for a class of six residents [2–6].

In 2013, the average United States Medical Licensing Examination® (USMLE®) score for matched US Seniors was 240 on Step 1 and 242 on Step 2, whereas unmatched US Seniors averaged 211 and 214 on USMLE scores, respectively. A candidate generally needs at least a 220 to be considered competitive, with other factors coming into play when extending interview invitations. According to the 2012 NRMP *Program Director Survey*, the most important factors used when ranking applicants for radiology residency were interactions during the interview, medical school performance, and perceived commitment to the specialty.

QUICK FACTS

Rank: Competitive
Median salary: $459 186
Residency years: 5 years (including Preliminary)
Number of residency positions: 1143 (164 PGY-1 and 979 PGY-2)
Number of filled residency positions: 1078 (94.3%)
Number filled by US Seniors: 825 (72.2%)
Number of applicants for PGY-2:
  US Seniors: 865
  Total: 1307
Median number of applications:
  US Seniors: 45
  Independent: 50
Median number of interviews offered:
  US Seniors: 20
  Independent: 8
Median number of programs ranked:
  US Seniors: 14
  Independent: 7
Average resident work hours: 40–50 hours
Average attending work hours: 50 hours
Resident call: In-house
Data based on [2–4]

Chapter 3

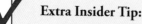

Extra Insider Tip:

- **The training pathway for IR is changing rapidly and moving towards being a distinct residency program.** Be sure to inquire how a residency program plans to respond to the new certification demands – this is important whether or not you are going into IR, because losing a fellow resident at the start of the 4th year may affect your call schedule.

- **The interview and everything associated with it is extremely important.** The interview is perhaps the most important factor in determining whether you will match at a program. Radiology residents spend a large amount of time interacting with attending radiologists at the workstation and during procedures. The ideal resident has an outgoing personality, but is also intelligent and conscientious. On interview day, try to convey these characteristics. Be enthusiastic and engaging, but be careful not to appear strange or insincere. Over the last few application cycles, we have had several instances of residents with excellent qualifications on paper being ranked low because of odd, seemingly contrived acts such as unwavering eye contact or progressively moving closer to an interviewer. We strongly recommend filtering out these behaviors through several mock interviews at your home institution.

- **If offered, go to the dinner the night before the interview, but make sure to be professional!** Your interactions with the residents are just as important as your actual interview. During the interview day, we always ask our residents about their interactions with the candidates. Even the suggestion of unusual conduct can devastate an applicant's chances. Not attending the dinner also carries negative connotations, but if you feel uncomfortable in these types of social situations, there is no reason to highlight this trait. It is probably better to limit your interactions to interview day.

- **Take USMLE Step 2 if your Step 1 scores are low.** We receive approximately 700 applications to fill 10 residency slots. Our admissions teams review applications with Step 1 scores above 230. The remaining applications are briefly reviewed by one of the Program Directors. Occasionally, those with lower USMLE Step 1 scores are given interviews, but usually only if their Step 2 scores are significantly higher. Candidates successfully matching at a highly competitive residency program often have USMLE Step 1 scores above 250.

- **If you go to a national meeting for networking, consider attending the Association of University Radiologists (AUR) annual meeting.** Many medical students go to RSNA, which is a large national meeting held yearly in Chicago with more than 50 000 attendees, but it is easy to get lost in the shuffle. Instead, consider attending the much smaller AUR meeting, where there are a large number of Program Directors.

- **Visit www.auntminnie.com during the interview process.** The medical student forums alert applicants of interview day options that residency programs are offering. They also allow for communication among applicants if you are interested in switching interview days, but be wary of working outside a program coordinator's scheduling efforts.

- **Consider applying for awards/grants.** Those specific to radiology include the Radiology Society of North America Research Medical Student Grant. The Association of University Radiologists offers the AMSER Henry Goldberg and Memorial Awards.

References

1. ABR: Interventional Radiology/Diagnostic Radiology (IR/DR) – Latest Information; available from: http://www.theabr.org/sites/all/themes/abr-media/pdf/ABR-IR-DR-FAQ.pdf [accessed March 2014].

2. NRMP (2013) *Data Release and Research Committee: Results of the 2013 NRMP Applicant Survey by Preferred Specialty and Applicant Type.* Washington, DC: National Resident Matching Program.

3. NRMP (2013) *Results and Data: 2013 Main Residency Match®.* Washington, DC: National Resident Matching Program.

4. AMGA (2012) *Medical Group Compensation and Financial Survey.* Alexandria, VA: American Medical Group Association.

5. NRMP (2012) *Data Release and Research Committee: Results of the 2012 NRMP Applicant Survey by Preferred Specialty and Applicant Type.* Washington, DC: National Resident Matching Program.

6. NRMP (2011) *Charting Outcomes in the Match, 2011.* Washington, DC: National Resident Matching Program.

Chapter 3

Radiology Oncology

Sara Alcorn, MD, MPH and Stephanie Terezakis, MD
John Hopkins University School of Medicine, Baltimore, MD

Introduction

Radiation oncologists use ionizing radiation to treat malignancies and some benign disorders. Along with Medical and Surgical Oncology, Radiation Oncology is one of the three main specialties that manage cancer in the US, and radiotherapy is estimated to be indicated in the treatment of over half of all cases of cancer. Modalities of radiotherapy include external beam radiation, brachytherapy, and radioisotope therapy, often in combination with surgical and chemotherapeutic treatments.

Modern Radiation Oncology involves the use of imaging modalities including ultrasound, X-ray, computed tomography (CT), positron emission tomography (PET), and magnetic resonance imaging (MRI) to identify and develop radiotherapy plans focused on a treatment target. This requires radiation oncologists to translate cross-sectional imaging into three-dimensional volumes, and thus the field favors physicians with excellent spatial reasoning skills. Radiation oncologists also must have a comprehensive understanding of anatomy in order to optimally focus radiotherapy plans on the treatment target while minimizing radiation exposure to nearby normal tissues.

Among the most technology-based specialties, radiation oncologists are often attracted to the fast-paced technological advances that characterize radiotherapy. This also requires adaptability and dedication to life-long learning, as radiation oncologists must adapt their practice to reflect evolving technologies.

Radiation Oncology is an evidence-based specialty that places a high premium on research. The field has the highest proportion of MD-PhD applicants of all specialties, with 22% of matched applicants carrying this dual degree [1]. Further, because cancer management has increasingly come to involve multiple treatment modalities, radiation oncologists must be well acquainted with the literature supporting best practices among other oncology specialties and skilled at integrating these diverse – and at times conflicting – data for clinical decision making.

On the other hand, our day-to-day work is characterized by frequent and often intense interactions with patients. Thus, residencies are looking for the whole package: applicants who, in addition to clinical knowledge and research contributions, have superb interpersonal skills and who prioritize delivery of compassionate care to our patients.

Including a Preliminary Year, Radiation Oncology residency is 5 years in duration. A minority (13%) of programs offers residency spots that include a Preliminary Year; the remainder of spots are filled as PGY-2 positions [2]. Many programs offer research time that can supplant clinical responsibilities for interested residents; this is generally done during the second half of residency, for up to 1 year. Some programs participate in the Holman Pathway offered through the American Board of Radiology, which grants residents up to 21 months of research time. Fellowships following residency are available in areas such as Proton Therapy, Brachytherapy, and Pediatrics. However, doing a fellowship remains relatively uncommon and is not generally required for employment.

Insider Tip: For each program, make sure you find out the amount of research time, if any, available to residents and whether both clinical and basic research endeavors are supported.

Primarily an outpatient specialty, most residents work closely with one or two attending in specialized subsites (such as genitourinary or breast cancer) for blocks of time, generally ranging from 1 to 4 months. Inpatient interactions are typically limited to urgent call cases and occasional discussions with inpatients with a new diagnosis of cancer.

Resident workload and expectations vary significantly by program. Some Radiation Oncology departments are seeing increasingly higher volumes. Nevertheless, since Radiation Oncology is largely an outpatient field, residents have nights and weekends without hospital responsibilities aside from occasional call. However, most residents spend significant time outside of the hospital studying, preparing for clinic, and participating in research projects. All programs are required to provide lectures covering clinical topics, as well as classes in radiation physics and radiation biology.

Preparation

Pre-Clinical Years

Excellent preparation in the basic sciences will provide a basis for understanding the complex concepts of cancer biology. Learning and retaining gross anatomy will serve as a building block for future radiotherapy treatment planning. As with any competitive specialty, applicants should aim to perform well on United States Medical Licensing Examination® (USMLE®) Steps 1 and 2.

Clinical Years

Applicants should strive for the highest grades in all clinical rotations, paying particular attention to Medicine, Surgery, and Pediatrics. Rotations in Radiology and Medical Oncology are also useful preparation.

At least one rotation in Radiation Oncology is required, preferably at your home institution if possible. An away rotation at another institution is highly recommended. However, keep in mind that doing an away rotation at one of your top choices can be risky and you will need to make every effort to leave your rotation having made a memorably positive impression should you be interested in matching at the program. Applicants without Radiation Oncology residencies at their home institution will need to be especially proactive in finding away rotations and establishing mentorship there.

Insider Tip: During rotations, you will not be expected to know much about the specifics of radiotherapy, but you will be evaluated closely on how well your personality meshes with that of the program. The best impressions are left by those who come across as personable, hard-working team players. A good fund of knowledge can be very impressive, but it must be communicated appropriately.

Chapter 3

Insider Tip: Do not be afraid to ask for letters of recommendation (LoRs) from the Chair and/or Program Director during your home and away rotations – they expect it! As they regularly have to write letters for students after only a few days in clinic together, be prepared to provide your résumé.

Involvement in research should be considered an unwritten requirement for matching into Radiation Oncology. US applicants who matched have an average of 8.3 abstracts, presentations, and publications, with even higher numbers reported among independent applicants [1]. Becoming involved in meaningful research requires establishing an early relationship with a mentor – the earlier, the better. The topic of your research does not need to be directly related to Radiation Oncology. However, having a radiation oncologist as a research mentor is extremely helpful, as he/she can be among your greatest allies and may go to bat for you during the application process. Also, research within Radiation Oncology further proves that you have sufficient exposure and commitment to the specialty.

Insider Tip: When looking for a research mentor, a good place to start is by searching for common interests among the faculty biographies usually found on departmental websites. Also, the chief or other current residents will be able to give you advice on which attendings or researchers are most amendable to working with medical students and who has available projects up for grabs.

Insider Tip: When you first meet with the researcher, you usually do not need to have a specific project in mind. Instead expect to highlight some of your mutual areas of interest and ask the researcher what projects are currently in the works. In most cases, if they have agreed to meet with you, they will have something in mind for you!

How much research is enough? The average US applicant who matches in Radiation Oncology reports 4.2 research experiences. Although it is very rare for an applicant with no research experience to be selected for a competitive residency spot, 85% of applicants who report only one or two research experiences still match into Radiation Oncology [1]. It is increasingly common for applicants with little research experience to take time off to build up their research résumés, commonly between the third and fourth years of medical school or after fourth year but prior to applying for residency. Alternatively, some medical schools have masters programs, such as in public health, which can be done between the third and fourth years and may allow time for research.

> ✓ **Insider Tip:** Submit an abstract to an annual meeting such as the American Society for Radiation Oncology (ASTRO), American Radium Society (ARS), or American Society of Clinical Oncology (ASCO). Attending these conferences is a great way to network, and posters and presentations help to beef up your research résumé – especially since you may not have your work published by the time that residency applications are due.

Residencies are looking for well-rounded, social applicants who will increase departmental diversity. As such, extracurricular activities that are unique or display leadership skills should be pursued. Moreover, such activities often are good discussion points during interviews.

> ✓ **Insider Tip:** When in doubt regarding the quality of your résumé, ask to meet with the residency Program Director where you do your Radiation Oncology rotation. This person is in the best position to offer advice regarding the competitiveness of your application and what you can do to improve your chances of matching. Meet with your Program Director early in your medical school career if you have interest in the field, particularly since it takes time to accrue good research experiences.

Applying

In 2013, 183 Radiation Oncology positions were offered, consisting of 160 PGY-2 spots and 23 PGY-1 spots (with combined Preliminary Years); 96% of these potential positions were filled. Of these, 83% were filled by US Seniors. International Medical Graduates (IMGs) filled 2.2% of the total spots. In 2011, among matched US Seniors, 31.2% were members of Alpha Omega Alpha, 22.2% had PhD degrees, and 7.8% had another type of graduate degree. The mean USMLE Step 1 and 2 scores were 240 and 244, respectively, and matched applicants reported an average of 8.3 abstracts/presentations/publications, 4.2 research experiences, 2.2 work experiences, and 5.9 volunteer experiences. These figures were slightly higher among independent seniors who matched [1–4].

QUICK FACTS

Rank: Highly competitive
Median salary: $471 000
Residency years: 5 years (including Preliminary)
Number of residency positions: 183 (23 PGY1 and 160 PGY2)
Number of filled residency positions: 176 (96%)
Number filled by US Seniors: 151 (83%)
Number of applicants for PGY-2:
  US Seniors: 170
  Total: 211
Median number of applications:
  US Seniors: 56
  Independent: 63
Median number of interviews offered:
  US Seniors: 16
  Independent: 6
Median number of programs ranked:
  US Seniors: 12
  Independent: 6
Average resident work hours: 40–50 hours
Average attending work hours: 40 hours
Resident call: Home call
Data based upon [2, 4, 5]

Chapter 3

Insider Tip: Do not panic! Remember that despite the daunting statistics above, nearly 80% of all US Seniors who applied for PGY-2 positions matched in 2013. However, this number is significantly higher than the 46% for independent applicants.

Among surveyed Radiation Oncology Program Directors, the five factors most frequently cited as important in selecting applicants for interviews were LoRs in the specialty, the personal statement, the USMLE/Comprehensive Osteopathic Medical Licensing Examination of the United States (COMLEX-USA®) Step 1 score, demonstration of involvement and interest in research, and perceived commitment to the specialty [3]. Although USMLE Step 1 and 2 scores tend to not be as highly prioritized in Radiation Oncology as in other similarly competitive specialties, a number of programs use minimum Step 1 scores to weed out potential interviewees. Of 25 surveyed programs, the USMLE Step 1 score below which they generally did not offer interviews ranged from 200 to 225 (median 220) [3]. Applicants concerned about their USMLE Step 1 scores should plan to take Step 2 in time for the application process.

Interviews

An incredibly important factor used to rank residents is their performance at the interview [3]. Keep in mind that you will be evaluated during all aspects of the interview process – including your interactions with office assistants, fellow interviewees, and residents – before, during, and after the interview. Personable applicants who seem like team players will be ranked higher than applicants who come off as arrogant, regardless of the rest of their résumés. Our field is very small, and most residents and faculty from different programs know each other and are friendly. Be aware that you should always be courteous and honest to everyone you meet on the interview trail, because it is very likely you will interact with them in the future.

Although the format varies, generally you should expect to have interviews with the Program Director, Department Chair, the chief or another resident, and often other clinical and research faculty. Usually these are one-on-one, but occasionally programs use pairs or panels of interviewers. The interview process at larger programs may take place over 2 days.

Insider Tip: If your medical school offers mock interview sessions, participate! If not, find a faculty mentor, current Radiation Oncology resident, or at least a classmate to practice interview questions with you.

Insider Tip: Do some research ahead of time. For each program, review the departmental website, and read the biographies of faculty members and residents, if available. This will give you a sense of the projects and research unique to the institution. Make a list of questions – and try to match these to relevant potential interviewers.

Extra Insider Tip:
- The **Association of Residents in Radiation Oncology (ARRO)** is an excellent resource for medical students and residents alike. Additional useful tips can be found on the ARRO website: https://www.astro.org/ARRO/Future-Residents/Index.aspx.

References

1. NRMP (2011) *Charting Outcomes in the Match, 2011*. Washington, DC: National Resident Matching Program.
2. NRMP (2013) *Results and Data: 2013 Main Residency Match®*. Washington, DC: National Resident Matching Program.
3. NRMP (2012) *Data Release and Research Committee: Results of the 2012 NRMP Program Director Survey*. Washington, DC: National Resident Matching Program.
4. NRMP (2013) *Data Release and Research Committee: Results of the 2013 NRMP Program Director Survey*. Washington, DC: National Resident Matching Program.
5. AMGA (2012) *Medical Group Compensation and Financial Survey*. Alexandria, VA: American Medical Group Association.

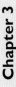

Chapter 3

Urology

Michael Granieri, MD and Andrew C. Peterson, MD, FACS
Duke University Medical Center, Durham, NC

Introduction

Urology is a unique specialty in its utilization of medical, endoscopic, and surgical therapy to treat a variety of disease processes among patients of all ages. Therefore, the successful urologist must have a strong combination of keen academic acumen, excellent hand–eye coordination, and the ability to adapt to evolving technologies. This breadth of requirements can make training challenging but also rewarding, as one can easily find a niche within the specialty. A Urology resident will treat not only a variety of genitourinary cancers across all ages and genders (bladder, kidney, prostate, testicular), but also benign disease process with significant quality of life issues (erectile dysfunction, voiding dysfunction, kidney stones, male factor infertility).

Not every Urology residency program is the same. The format and length of training vary, but is a minimum of 5 years. Many programs consist of a Preliminary Year of General Surgery (internship) followed by 4 years of Clinical Urology. There are rare programs that offer 2 years of General Surgery with 3 years of Urology. Others are 6 years long, offering an integrated year of Urology research (usually in year 4). Candidates should determine which of these is right for them and select programs accordingly.

Once training is completed, graduates may enter directly into practice or pursue subspecialty fellowships in Urologic Oncology, Minimally Invasive Surgery, Pediatric Urology, Andrology, Female Urology, or Trauma/Reconstruction. These fellowships typically range from 1 to 2 years.

Resident's View

Due to its surgical nature, Urology residency can be both time-consuming and challenging. Days typically start at 6:30 a.m. and end around 6 p.m., sometimes longer. The workload greatly depends on your training program, call schedule, and operative volume. However, your day does not end when you leave the hospital, as Urology residents need to prepare for the following day's cases, conferences, or clinic.

Call schedules vary greatly, with some programs having transitioned to a night-float system that emphasizes shift work and limits weekend call responsibility. However, many programs still have the traditional "home call," which can vary in time and work required depending on the number of hospitals covered.

Despite all of these challenges, the majority of Urology residents have more free time to pursue their out-of-hospital interests and responsibilities than many of their surgical counterparts. Therefore, we think that Urology residents tend to be very satisfied with their career choice.

Preparation

Program Director's View

Urology faculty and Program Directors generally are looking for applicants who have demonstrated an early interest in Urology. However, faculty and Program Directors understand that exposure to this specialty early in medical school is often limited, so that some applicants will be "latecomers" to the Urology application process. Therefore, it is imperative to have demonstrated an early interest in one of the procedural specialties (e.g., General Surgery, Orthopedic Surgery). Therefore, we recommend students interact frequently with mentors in medical school to help guide them in their early experiences.

Specific areas in which applicant review committees prioritize include performance on clinical rotations (Junior Surgery clerkship, Urology subinternships), letters of recommendations (LoRs) from surgical mentors/supervisors, experience in surgically oriented research (while research in urology is recommended, research in any surgical field is helpful), grades in medical school, and (very importantly) standardized testing scores on the United States Medical Licensing Examination® (USMLE®) series.

Insider Tip: Do not delay taking USMLE Step 2. Program Directors may take this as an indication that you are not confident in your ability to score well.

Resident's View

Applying to Urology can be daunting because of limited exposure during medical school, the early match process, and the small number of residency positions. In addition, Urology applicants are among the best and brightest medical students, making competition tough!

There are many ways to succeed in the match process, but early preparation is helpful. This means pursuing a Urology elective early in your third year to determine if the field is right for you. If so, early involvement in research can really bolster an application by demonstrating a genuine interest in the field and allowing you to work closely with Urology faculty. The latter is critical, because in such a small field, LoRs (that are usually accrued during these rotations) carry more weight than in other specialties.

However, many programs recognize the aforementioned challenges and thus seek out applicants who have not only performed exceptionally well during their clinical rotations and USMLE examinations, but also demonstrated success in other extracurricular activities. Although not essential, one should strive to be in the top 25% of the class with a USMLE Step 1 score above 230.

Chapter 3

Applying

Program Director's View

Our program is interested in the well-rounded applicant; those with outstanding test scores, good grades in medical school, excellent LoRs, evidence of prior active research, and a personality that will fit into our program. The faculty tend to concentrate on grades, LoRs, and test scores while the residents have different areas of concern (see below). While the entire application is evaluated, some programs have USMLE cutoffs that vary by program.

QUICK FACTS

Rank: Highly competitive
Average salary: $415 598
Residency years: 5 years (including Preliminary)
Number of residency positions: 285
Number of filled residency positions: 285 (100%)
Number of applicants: 446
   Matched: 285
   Unmatched: 161
Average number of applications: 59
Average number of interviews offered: 10
Average resident work hours: 60–80
Average attending work hours: 50–60 hours
Resident call: Program-dependent
Data based upon [1, 2]

In 2014, 285 Urology positions were offered and 100% of these positions were filled. There were a total of 446 applicants, 161 of whom did not match, resulting in approximately 1.6 applicants per position. Clearly Urology is a highly competitive specialty. The average applicant submitted 59 applications and received 10 interview offers; 68% of US Seniors were successful in matching and 24% of International Medical Graduates (IMGs) found a position [1, 2].

Resident's View

The first step is to meet with your Urology Department's Medical Student Advisor to get a sense of your competitiveness. Once this is established, apply to a broad list of programs. Most applicants apply to about 45–60 programs, but this varies depending on your geographical preferences, career goals, and competitiveness. Your advisor can help you identify programs that may be a good fit. The www.urologymatch.com website is also a great resource and is very popular among Urology applicants.

 Insider Tip: Interview at about 15 programs. To meet this goal, it is best to "over apply" and then cancel interviews rather than "under apply" and risk being offered less than 15 interviews.

 Insider Tip: Your personal statement should be a thoughtful, well-written story of how you chose Urology, but in most cases it will not significantly impact your chances of getting an interview.

 Insider Tip: Urology is a very small, close-knit community, so that strong LoRs from well-known faculty can make a significant positive impact on your application.

Interview Day

Program Director's View

From the faculty's perspective, once applicants haves made it through the vetting process and been selected for an interview, they are considered to be finalists. The interview is one of our final steps in the selection process. During interview day, the specific components being addressed include professionalism, interpersonal skills and communication, appearance, personality and charm, and, very importantly the ability to fit seamlessly into the program. It is extremely important for the applicant to interact appropriately with fellow residents and faculty.

In order to better assess this, we have designed our interview day to include a "residents-only" pre-interview dinner, tour of the facilities, and interviews with multiple key clinical faculty and current residents. We believe it is important for the residents to have significant input because they will be working on a daily basis with matched applicants. We look closely at the applicant's behavior and ability to interact in both informal situations (the dinner the night before) as well as in formal and sometimes stressful situations (the scheduled interviews).

Insider Tip: Program Directors and faculty are looking for people who are not only honest, interesting, and fun to be around, but also outgoing and professional. This is where the "residents-only" pre-interview dinner is very important, because we are able to compare an applicant's personality in these informal situations to the formalized interview process.

Insider Tip: Be familiar with the program on interview day. Look up the program's website and know about the rotation schedule, strengths in research, and clinical experience of the program. This will allow you to ask thoughtful and insightful questions.

Insider Tip: If you go to a national meeting, attend the American Urological Association (AUA) Meeting. Having presentations at this meeting either on the podium or in poster sessions increases your visibility to Program Directors and faculty.

Resident's View

We emphasize personality and program "fit." We typically are not privy to the details of the application (if you got this far, you are academically capable), but rather evaluate your personality, interpersonal communication skills, and overall likeability. With so many excellent applicants, many times this involves splitting hairs. However, sometimes applicants show "red flags" that make our job easier. These include being rude to residents, faculty, other applicants,

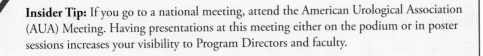

Chapter 3

or support staff; drinking too much at the pre-interview dinner; disheveled appearance; or being late to interview events without giving prior notice.

For the actual interviews, you should be prepared to talk about *anything* on your application, including any and all prior research. It is important to appear relaxed yet engaged, smiling appropriately and showing interest in the program by asking questions. It is your time to learn as much about the program as they will about you.

> **Insider Tip:** Spend time getting to know the residents at each program. This is the best way to get a feel for the program's culture and whether you would be a good fit.

Summary

Matching into Urology is challenging but rewarding. Your first priority should be performing well in your clerkships and scoring well on USMLE Step 1. Once you have decided Urology is the right career for you, it is in your best interest to meet with your department's Student Advisor, engage in research projects, and perform well on your subinternships. This will bolster your application and strengthen LoRs, which can make a big difference in a small field. During the interview process, it is best to be polite, likeable, and friendly with everybody you meet (not just on interview day!).

> **Extra Insider Tips:**
> - **Visit www.urologymatch.com.** This is the urologist's equivalent to student–doctor network. You will find a wealth of useful information on this website, such as a residency guide, discussion forum, and program reviews.
> - **Visit www.auanet.org.** This is the official site of the American Urologic Association. In the education section you can find helpful study materials, listings of all the accredited Urology programs, and a timeline for the match process.

References

1. AMGA (2012) *Medical Group Compensation and Financial Survey.* Alexandria, VA: American Medical Group Association.
2. American Urologic Association; available from: http://www.auanet.org/education/urology-and-specialty-matches.cfm [accessed June 2014].

Chapter 3

4: Path to the Match

Medical students are veritable linear thought machines. Following sequential steps to their logical conclusion is a method that has been perpetuated since kindergarten. However, linear processes pose the threat of being both rigid and time-consuming. This is especially true in the path to the Match. Too often, medical students focus solely on grades in the pre-clinical years, then move on to United States Medical Licensing Examination® (USMLE®) Step 1, then core third-year rotations, then specialty choice, and, lastly, residency program selection (Figure 4.1). They take everything one step at a time, as they have been so diligently taught.

> **Insider Tip:** *WRONG way to approach medical school* – Medical school is not simply linear steps to accomplish before graduation.

In reality, by the time the third year ends, you will have completed 90% of the required elements of your residency application. Hopefully, you will have plans to finish the remaining 10% by October 1, the date of the Medical School Performance Evaluation (MSPE) release. With this short time frame, the path to a *successful* match cannot be linear, lest you risk making a hurried, uninformed, and ill-prepared decision about one of the most important aspects of your future. In recognition of the utility of non-linear medical education, some schools have abandoned the idea of a curriculum of pre-clinical followed by clinical years, instead adopting vertical integration of the classroom and clinical experience [1,2]. If your school has not caught up to this latest pedagogic trend, it is up to you to acquire the exposure you need to make the right specialty choice. It may mean spending personal time such as weekends, spring break, or possibly that coveted "last summer" between first and second year of medical school shadowing a physician or performing specialty-specific research. These experiences not only allow you the opportunity to explore career options, but also build residency application fodder and professional contacts.

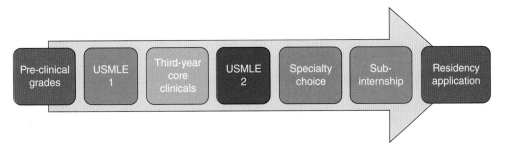

Figure 4.1 Typical approach to medical school.

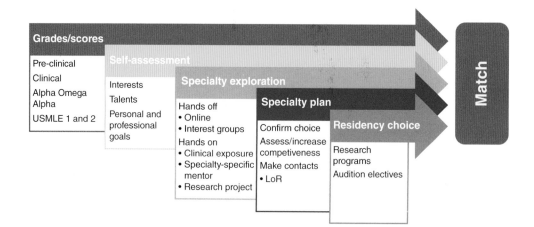

Figure 4.2 A different approach to medical school.

As early as possible, begin to think of the medical school curriculum, specialty choice, and residency program selection as overlapping processes leading towards the residency match. Figure 4.2 provides a brief overview of this concept, with the steps of self-assessment and specialty exploration and selection discussed in more detail in the previous chapters. The current chapter explains how to prioritize your curricular and extracurricular medical school activities and accomplishments in relation to your eventual residency application. If you are reading this book in your pre-clinical years, that is great! It demonstrates an early understanding of medical school as a time to not only learn the material, but also prepare for your future career. We will help you along that journey. If you are reading this book in your clinical years, no need to panic – it is not too late! You likely have already undertaken some of the preparatory steps without even realizing it. With the Match just around the corner, we will teach you how to highlight what you have achieved thus far, while focusing your efforts in the time that remains to effectively bolster your application.

 Insider Tip: *RIGHT way to approach medical school* – Your true medical education is a series of overlapping steps designed to not only teach you the material, but also allow adequate specialty exploration and preparation for a successful residency match and eventually a career.

Selection Process and Board Scores

In order to work productively towards a residency position of your choice, you need to understand the selection process. This will be discussed in greater detail and with more insider advice in the following chapter. For now, we will provide you with a basic frame of reference to better navigate the path to the Match.

The information you input into the Electronic Residency Application System (ERAS®) will essentially generate a résumé, or as we call it in the academic world, a curriculum vitae (CV), which describes your educational, research, and extracurricular endeavors. Other documents in your ERAS application folder include a medical school transcript, MSPE, United States Medical Licensing Examination® (USMLE®) or Comprehensive Osteopathic Medical Licensing Examination of the United States (COMLEX-USA®) transcripts, personal statement, letters of recommendation (LoRs), and a photograph.

USMLE

While there is some variation among programs, many residency programs perform an initial filter of all residency applicants based on a quantitative measure – the USMLE Step 1 score. Where exactly that cutoff USMLE score is set is determined by the competitiveness of the program and specialty. At times, the cutoff can be difficult to discern. Some programs may post the minimum score on their website. For those that do not, you can find the average accepted scores in the National Resident Matching Program (NRMP®)'s *Charting Outcomes in the Match* [3], and estimate the requisite score based on the program's reputation and the caliber of residents currently in attendance (check the program's online resident profile). Another option is to scan medical student chat forums. These are usually rife with applicants' interview invitations paired with their USMLE scores, but be aware that there is no way to be sure that the information provided is accurate or up-to-date.

Appreciating the fact that a board score does not encapsulate you as a medical student, there will likely be one or more secondary reviewers who assess the remaining pieces of your application for other attractive features. Whether all other applications, or just those with a USMLE Step 1 score slightly lower than the cutoff, are reviewed depends on the program. However, as this is a time-consuming process, this secondary review may basically be an expanded quantitative screen, focusing on USMLE Step 2 scores, grades, and Alpha Omega Alpha status. Therefore, an increasing number of schools are advising their students to take USMLE Step 2, particularly CK (Clinical Knowledge), early enough to be considered in their application. In fact, some residency programs require it for application so be sure to check the individual program websites. At the time of the 2013 NRMP Match, 80% of applicants had taken USMLE Step 2 CK [3]. In 2012, the NRMP surveyed residency Program Directors to ascertain the factors used in selecting applicants for interview and ranking. USMLE Step 1 scores received the highest number of votes for granting interviews, with 82% of Program Directors citing it as an important factor [4]. USMLE Step 2 scores received 70% of Program Director votes, which is even more than those listing grades in the clerkship of the desired specialty as influential (69%) [4]. While USMLE Step 1 scores assess a student's mastery of the basic sciences, Step 2 scores are a measure of a student's ability to apply that knowledge to patient care. USMLE Step 2 CK is a 1-day, computer-based examination, whereas Step 2 CS (Clinical Skills) uses standardized patients to test physical examination and patient communication skills. The notoriously high pass rate for the USMLE Step 2 CS component makes it less useful as a criterion for interview selection.

Chapter 4

Your secondary quantitative measures may put you on the interview list. However, if you are still teetering on the cusp, qualitative measures such as your personal statement and LoRs can tip you over in either direction. Nevertheless, if you were still a "maybe" at this secondary stage of review, these documents would have to be very impressive in order to garner an interview. Examples include a LoR from a leader in the field saying you are the best and brightest he/she has ever worked with or a personal statement that practically brings tears to the eyes of a reader.

Once you pass the initial screen and are granted an interview, these quantitative measurements alone will not be enough to ensure a residency position. At interview time, your interviewer will likely (though not always) take a closer look at your application. This review often is as much about "appraising your worth" as it is about finding discussion points for the interview. At this juncture, research and extracurricular interests, as well as a well-written and interesting personal statement, can be a great advantage. Shortly after, if not at the end of your interview day, all interviewers will meet and rank that day's applicants in relation to the other applicants they have met thus far. When two applicants are being considered for the same rank position, quantitative assessments may be used as a tie breaker. However, it is often an interviewer's subjective experience of the interaction that decides how an applicant is eventually ranked. It is not at all uncommon for a person with fantastic scores/grades to appear arrogant or robotic during an interview and subsequently be moved down the rank list. No attending wants to work alongside that person for the next few years. Sometimes a great personality and compelling extracurricular interest may move you further up the list than your scores would dictate. For example, one year we interviewed an applicant with average scores who was an accomplished underwater photographer. During the interview, he shared his photographs which had been on display at the Smithsonian. His description of how he spent hours creating these masterpieces clearly demonstrated an attention to detail and passion beyond the typical applicant. He obviously impressed many programs as he ended up matching at one of the most competitive programs in the country.

As you can see, all facets of your application and eventual interview play a part, but it is a solid USMLE score that can get you in the door. Getting an interview despite missing the initial USMLE Step 1 cutoff can be an uphill battle, but certainly is not impossible. If your scores are slightly below par for the residency program of your choice, you will have to work harder to make the other parts of your application shine.

COMLEX

COMLEX is the osteopathic equivalent to the allopathic USMLE, with similar content, temporal sequence, and structure. Levels 1, 2 (Level 2 is split into PE (Performance Evaluation) and CE (Cognitive Evaluation)), and 3 are usually administered in postgraduate years PGY-1, PGY-2, and PGY-4, respectively. All attendees of accredited osteopathic medical schools are eligible to take the COMLEX (American College of Graduate Medical Education (ACGME) medical school students are not). However, osteopathic medical school students are also eligible to take the USMLE and an increasing number are doing so. Cross-referencing the 2010 American Association of Colleges of Osteopathic Medicine (AACOM) graduate information available at the time of publication with the concurrent NRMP Match data reveals that 1444 of the total 3631 graduating osteopathic medical students (40%) matched into ACGME-accredited residency programs [3, 5]. The most common reason cited by osteopathic medical students for making the switch to an allopathic residency program is to "keep [their] options open" [6, 7]. Compared with osteopathic pathways, there are a larger number of ACGME residency programs, with a greater variety of specialization options. The ACGME accredits more than 9000 graduate medical education programs, which train approximately 116 000 resident physicians. In comparison, the American Osteopathic Association (AOA) accredits just over 1000 osteopathic graduate programs training 6900 resident physicians [8]. In terms of osteopathic subspecialization options, there are many that parallel those offered by ACGME programs. Refer to the AOA website (www.osteopathic.org) for a comprehensive list. However, some areas are under-represented or not represented at all. For instance, osteopathic medical students have fewer opportunities for surgical subspecialty training, as many of the osteopathic training programs were established in areas of primary care physician shortage with the express purpose of providing general care to rural and underserved populations [9]. Geographically, 83% of all AOA-approved residency positions are located within only 10 states. With geography cited as the top criterion by which fourth-year students choose residency locations [10], this predilection for osteopathic programs to be located in rural areas is another reason why a student may opt for an urban-based and/or larger allopathic institution.

Most ACGME-approved residency programs require USMLE Step 1 scores for applicants to their PGY-1 or categorical programs (admission to PGY-2 positions is a special issue that will be discussed below). Others are willing to accept COMLEX scores. However, even these programs may have misinformation or misgivings about the veracity of the conversion formulas translating COMLEX scores into the more familiar USMLE scores, limiting your potential to match into an allopathic program.

Whether or not an osteopathic student should take the USMLE is a somewhat controversial question. Some believe that it adds credence to the perception that the COMLEX is not an equivalent examination to the USMLE – "Why would you even want to go to a residency program that does not accept the COMLEX for consideration?" Others regard sitting for the USMLE with the obvious intent to go to an allopathic rather than osteopathic residency program as a rejection of the holistic osteopathic philosophy. Anecdotal reports of DO physicians who have taken ACGME residencies feeling ostracized by the osteopathic community led to the approval of Resolution B-14 by the AOA Bureau of Osteopathic Medical Educators requesting that "The AOA, its leaders, and its members should immediately cease referring to doctors of osteopathic medicine (DO) that completed a portion or all of their residency training in ACGME-accredited programs as 'having left the profession.' *Semper* DO … once a DO, always a DO" [11].

This debate recently has become even more contentious. In November 2011, the ACGME announced proposed changes to their Common Program Requirements that, as of 2014, would limit the access of DOs to advanced training and fellowship in programs approved by the ACGME (or Royal College of Physicians and Surgeons of Canada (RCPSC)) by requiring that a prerequisite preliminary training year or full residency, respectively, be limited to

Chapter 4

ACGME-accredited programs. Though this would not affect osteopathic students entering PGY-1 positions as categorical residents, it would greatly impact those who completed an AOA traditional rotating internship (TRI) as a PGY-1 with the plan to transfer into a PGY-2 categorical position or begin advanced training as a PGY-2 in those specialties that require 1 year of preliminary training (Anesthesiology, Dermatology, Diagnostic Radiology, Ophthalmology, Neurology, Physical Medicine and Rehabilitation, Psychiatry, Radiation Oncology, and Urology). This is especially problematic for those residing in one of the four states that require 1–2 years of an AOA TRI in order to obtain DO licensure, namely Florida, Maine, Michigan, and Pennsylvania. For residents of these states, there currently is an option to obtain a Resolution 42 waiver – a method of obtaining AOA approval of an ACGME-accredited PGY-1 and still qualify for DO licensure.

> **Insider Tip:** As an osteopathic medical student contemplating attending an allopathic residency program, be aware of the state-specific requirements for initial medical licensure (check Federation of State Medical Board (www.fsmb.org) in your desired practice location). Some states require 1–2 years of *osteopathic* postgraduate training in order to attain licensure.

The AOA recognized that, in view of these new Common Program Requirements, many students would abandon osteopathic residency programs if they were required to repeat their PGY-1 year or if they would later be denied access to ACGME fellowships. In March 2012, AOA and AACOM leadership met with ACGME officials to advocate amendment of the ACGME proposals. Initially, talks appeared promising, with all involved groups publically stating in October 2012 that they had entered into agreement to develop a Memorandum of Understanding (MOU) that would detail the process of a single unified accreditation system. However, by July 2013, it was announced that the groups could not agree on the MOU. While the details of the MOU rejection were not released, the AOA and AACOM cited a disagreement about the language of the draft proposed by the ACGME, rather than a dismissal of a unified accreditation system in its entirety. Over the next few months, the AOA reiterated their opposition to the Common Program Requirements [12]. However, in October 2013, the ACGME approved the initial proposed restrictions on AOA prerequisite training with two new additional provisions: (1) implementation of the approved changes would be delayed until July 2016 and (2) ACGME fellowship programs are allowed to select "exceptionally qualified applicants" who completed residency training in AOA-approved programs if they have taken and passed all levels of the USMLE [13].

Whatever your political viewpoints, it all boils down to your professional goals. If you want a career in family practice, you will have many osteopathic and even some allopathic residency options with a COMLEX score alone. If you wish to pursue a specialty with limited osteopathic resident or fellowship options via an ACGME program, a good USMLE score can help. However, note that this is a *good* score. While you are not required to divulge a bad

USMLE score as part of an ERAS application, you are required to state honestly whether or not you took the examination. Obviously, taking the examination and not releasing the result implies poor performance and either prospect will hurt your application. Those osteopathic students who take the USMLE Step 1 are faced with the same decision as allopathic students as to whether or not they should take Step 2 before applying. Passage of COMLEX Level 2-PE is required for graduation [14]. The idea of taking two extra examinations just for application purposes can be a major deterrent to osteopathic students. Of note, whether or not you receive a DO or MD license is determined by your medical school, not which licensing examination you take. Passage of the tri-level COMLEX is accepted for medical licensure in all 50 states; however, the ability to substitute the COMLEX with the USMLE in order to gain DO licensure is a state-specific issue. For instance, Oklahoma, Maine, Tennessee, California, and Arizona require passage of the COMLEX alone for licensure.

This is a very fluid time in healthcare, which is reflected in the rapidly changing requirements for residency and fellowship training. If you are an osteopathic student with an inclination toward ACGME postgraduate training at any level, you need to stay vigilant about the latest prerequisites, as there will likely be even more changes in the near future.

> **Insider Tip:** Recently approved changes to ACGME advanced residency and fellowship prerequisites restricting access to DO students have caused controversy and demands for change. If pursuing ACGME-accredited training, stay on top of the latest requirements.

Grades and Clinical Clerkship Schedule

Grades

You do not need a book to tell you that getting good grades is better than bad grades, so we will not insult your intelligence by including this as a tip. What we will do is point out that some grades matter more than others, particularly for certain specialties. If you are just starting out in medical school and have a notion of your ultimate specialty choice, this guide will tell you where to spend the bulk of your study time. If you are already preparing your application, this information will help you gauge your competitiveness. If you did well in the courses important to your specialty, try to subtly draw attention to that in a personal statement or interview. For example, you could note, "I first became interested in a surgical career during my anatomy course. I was drawn to and excelled in the precision of the technique, earning top marks in my class…"

If you happen to pursue a medical career in one of the basic sciences, such as pathology, obviously doing well in this as well as your other pre-clinical courses will be weighted more heavily than in other specialties. For instance, when the 2012 NRMP *Program Director Survey* respondents were asked to report the importance of various application factors on a 1–5 scale (least to most important), pathologists gave honors in the basic sciences an importance value of 3.5, whereas Program Directors in Emergency Medicine rated it as only 2.5 [4]. Other specialties single out specific pre-clinical courses, such as anatomy grades for applicants to Surgical residency, physiology for Anesthesiology, and microbiology for applicants to Internal Medicine residency who are planning to pursue a fellowship in Infectious Disease. The link between these courses and the specialty choice is clear, and should receive emphasis during study and application time.

However, across all specialties, performance in the required clinical and desired clinical clerkships are valued more than honors in the basic sciences, receiving 71, 69 and 45% of votes on the 2012 NRMP *Program Director Survey*, respectively [4]. To Program Directors, performance in clinical clerkships assesses your ability to assimilate book knowledge into patient care. Performance in the clerkship of your desired specialty is the closest approximation a Program Director has to assess your future performance as a resident.

Being prepared and knowledgeable about your patients is key to excelling in clinical rotations. Of course, many attendings will "pimp" you about a medical fact pertaining to your patient. In these instances, a solid background in the basic sciences will help, but by reading up on your patient's illness, you can anticipate these questions and shine. A large part of your evaluation will be determined by how succinctly you present the status of your patient and how readily you can answer questions about the patient's history and findings. A literature

Front

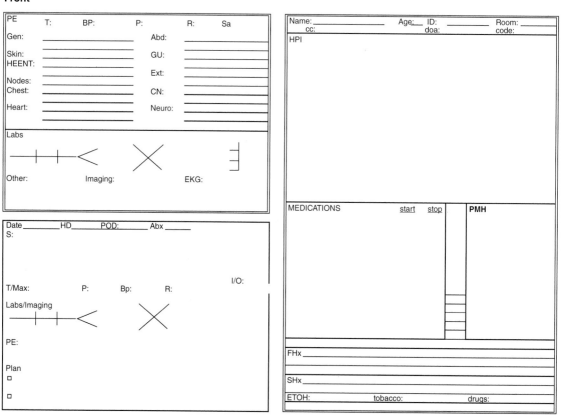

Figure 4.3 Sample patient tracker sheet.

review (2000–2009) searching for studies relating medical student personality traits to such performance indicators as academic prowess and clinical competence [15] reported that conscientiousness was a significant predictor of performance in medical school and became increasingly significant as students advanced through their clinical years. As a medical student on a clinical rotation, do all that is asked of you and then some. Always go that extra mile. As you become more adept with patient care and the intricacies of your current rotation, you will be able to work more efficiently by filtering out less important information about your patient. Until then, it is wise to carry a sheet with some (unidentified) vital patient facts such as history, medication, and laboratory values as well as a to-do list. Figure 4.3 is a sample patient tracker sheet. It was designed to be printed on the front and back of standard 8.5 × 11-inch paper and then folded over to fit comfortably in the pocket of a white coat.

Back:

Figure 4.3 (*Continued*)

> **Insider Tip:** A "conscientious" medical student is one who does well on his clinical rotations. Keep abreast of your patient's history, test results, and required tasks with a patient tracker similar to the sample provided.

Finally, Alpha Omega Alpha is an honor society to which membership is highly regarded by Program Directors, particularly in the more competitive programs and specialties. The local Alpha Omega Alpha chapter usually begins the process of selecting applicants based on grades and evidence of leadership and ethics, 16 months before a given class graduates. Some students are elected to membership in the spring of their third year (in time for applications); others are not chosen until graduation. Individual Alpha Omega Alpha chapters have substantial latitude in how they elect their members, so check with your Dean's Office about the requirements. There are very few medical schools without an Alpha Omega Alpha chapter, though these include such prestigious schools as Harvard and Stanford. Usually, this is because the school lacks a ranking system, has a pass/fail grading system (both class rank and grades are prerequisites for Alpha Omega Alpha), or students have voted against it. If this is the case, do not be concerned that lack of Alpha Omega Alpha membership will negatively affect your application as you will have the ability to indicate that Alpha Omega Alpha was not an option at your institution in the Profile section of your ERAS application.

Clerkship Schedule

The timing of your clinical clerkships is crucial. When starting your third year, if you are considering a career in one of the core clerkships, request to do that rotation early. This will give you time to pursue LoRs if it is the right fit or an opportunity to explore other options by the deadline for fourth-year schedule requests (usually spring of third year) if it is not. You may also want to consider doing a "warm-up" clerkship before a clerkship in your desired specialty in order to get used to being part of a clinical team and learn the ins and outs of the hospital, electronic medical record, and ordering system. For example, if contemplating a surgical career, it is probably wiser to do this rotation in the second half of the fall term after medicine. You will be much more efficient by that point, a much appreciated quality on a busy surgical service.

> **Insider Tip:** If scheduling allows, do a warm-up rotation before starting a clerkship in your desired specialty. You want to have made all your rookie mistakes on a rotation less important for your career.

If you already have a preferred residency program or geographic training location, consider taking an away elective at the end of your third year or the beginning of your fourth. This is paramount if you have negative attributes in your application, such as a subpar USMLE Step 1 score or if you have no clear regional ties to a program. Many times during a preliminary applicant screen or the post-interview applicant ranking process, a student who currently lives far way or has no family in the area is deemed someone "who will never come here." Programs consider it a feather in their cap if they do not drop too far down their rank list to fill all residency positions, so they will not waste a rank position on a candidate they think has no real intention of ranking them highly. These away electives are a chance for both you and the program to audition each other. If you are an extrovert with a solid work ethic, consider this an important opportunity to show the program that you would be a good fit. Many programs also grant what is known as a "courtesy interview" to those applicants who have done an away elective at their program. While it does not ensure a match, an outstanding performance will certainly move you up the rank list. Alternatively, there are two ways in which an audition elective can negatively impact your chances:

- Doing an away rotation in a program that is simply far too competitive for your grades and board scores. Away rotations are useful if you are on the edge of interview consideration. If you otherwise have zero chance of landing an interview at a residency program, in the absence of curing cancer while on service there, you will not be ranked high enough to match – courtesy interview or not. Focus your efforts on an achievable residency program.
- You are slightly introverted, or take a while to acclimate to new situations. A lackluster or unmemorable audition elective can seriously decrease your chances of being highly ranked at that program in the Match.

During your fourth year, there are other considerations integral to your clinical clerkship schedule. Through your Dean's Office, find out the date of the last course which will show up on your MSPE, usually early to mid September. Schedule your advanced rotations or subinternships before this deadline. A strong performance in these clerkships will boost your application. If you are planning on taking the advanced courses as a means of confirming a specialty choice or procuring a LoR, do them as early as possible. Once completing these courses, some applicants take a less strenuous rotation while compiling application materials. Others save these "breather rotations" for the interview period, which ranges from late October to early February depending on the specialty. Check residency program websites or specialty-specific student forums to get more detailed information about timing of interviews. Also check your school's policy regarding time off for interviews. While you are often provided a reasonable amount of interview time, you may find it too restrictive if you are attempting to increase chances of a match with a large number of interviews or if you are applying to more than one specialty, including Preliminary or Transitional programs. In that case, you may have to use vacation time for some of the allotted interviews.

After finally exhaling on Match Day, how you schedule your remaining months is up to you. Some students stick with less arduous rotations in order to be refreshed before starting the intern year. This is perfectly understandable. However, consider doing a rotation in an area that always interested you even if it does not relate to your career choice. You will never get another chance like this to explore a new area. As an alternative, consider taking a rotation in an area where you have had little exposure thus far but will become important during residency, such as the Intensive Care Unit, Anesthesia, or Emergency Medicine.

LoRs and Mentorship

LoRs reflect not only your accomplishments but also your ability to form meaningful relationships with faculty. Flattering letters written by attendings indicate that they were both impressed by your work and *liked* you. That is exactly what Program Directors want in their residents. The ideal LoR is highly complimentary and comes from a well-respected physician who knows you beyond a superficial level. As such, the sooner you can begin to cultivate these relationships, the better. Unfortunately, many students do not begin to make professional contacts until the clinical years and even then are very hesitant to reach out. In the pre-clinical years, most students have not settled on a specialty choice. They feel that time spent shadowing, researching or meeting with attendings who may be outside their ultimate specialty will be a wasted effort for all involved parties. However, this could not be further from the truth. Any time spent in a clinical or academic setting with a physician is an opportunity to confirm or eliminate that specialty as a potential choice. This is crucial to making the right career decision. The time spent could lead to an excellent recommendation and a glowing letter from a physician outside your field is still a wonderful addition to your application. Moreover, these attendings may have ties with your desired residency program or to physicians in your field. An informal phone call from them can open doors to a sought-after residency position or connect you with a potential specialty-specific mentor.

Hopefully, we have persuaded you to form relationships with faculty early, even if they are outside your field. The question is how to go about it. The place to start is the advisor your school likely assigned you upon matriculation. If you are one of the few students who knew your future specialty from day 1, you can request to be paired with an advisor in that department. If not, these relationships are still useful. Advisors are generally selected because they are enthusiastic about guiding medical students and are knowledgeable about the residency application process. Besides helping you navigate ERAS, they can give you information about the qualifications of former residency applicants who successfully matched and point you in the direction of faculty who have written laudatory LoRs in the past. The specialty mentors you seek out, while enthusiastic, may not be as up-to-date on the application process. Therefore, it is advantageous to have both types of advisors in your corner.

In addition to your advisor's recommendations for a specialty-specific mentor, you can do a little research on the attendings at your current or desired institution. Start with their online faculty profile. It usually lists where they trained, their research interests, and publications. If publications are not listed, query their name in the PubMed database and you will be able to discern their research focus. If your interests align, email them to see whether they are taking on research assistants, or if they would be willing to oversee a project of yours. "Knowing the players," is also a good tool when beginning clinical clerkships; it can help you procure an influential LoR or an interesting research project. Also, be mindful of where the attending trained. If it is a program you are considering, you are in luck, since they may still have ties to faculty there.

Upperclassmen as well as residents and faculty to whom you are exposed during your clinical years can also give advice about whom to approach for mentorship. Be sure to convey excitement about the field (though delicately if it is different than their own) and a willingness to work hard. No one wants to saddle a colleague with a lazy, dispassionate medical student. You are unlikely to get much assistance by nonchalantly asking, "I need to do research. Who is good?" as you leave early for the day.

If you are pursuing a specialty with few options for mentorship at your current institution, do not hesitate to go outside its walls. You can consider larger hospitals in the area or seek out attendings in your desired residency program or geographic location. Again, peruse faculty web pages for a potential match and email them, or ask your advisors to help connect you. Alumni are alternative resources for mentorship outside your current faculty. There may be an alumni association in place at your school. If not, request a list from your Dean's Office and start reaching out. In addition, many specialty- or medically-oriented political societies allow free student membership. Potential advisors can be found by attending specialty conferences or through the "Find a mentor in your area" programs that many specialty societies offer.

CV Fortification

Remember that your CV is your academic résumé. Besides listing your training, it also catalogues your research, presentations, publications, society memberships, extracurricular activities, and any work or other experience you may have had. Be sure to include this last aspect, especially if it explains a gap in your education. See also Chapter 8: *The Curriculum Vitae*.

Research

Ways to become involved in a research project were discussed in the LoR section of this chapter. However, there are several other points to be made about research as it pertains to your application. In the pre-clinical years, research can be a tool not only for buffing your CV, but also specialty exploration. The concern many students have about taking on a research project at this early stage is that you may have many, possibly divergent, career paths in mind and that research in an area which is not your end specialty choice is pointless. It is important to know, however, that many Program Directors value research in any field, especially if it is successful and has culminated in a manuscript or national presentation. However, if you have these concerns, consider a project that can be linked to several specialties or has an overarching role in the medical field. For instance, projects that encourage multidisciplinary training or patient care, a medical school education initiative, a quality assurance project, or medical informatics development, demonstrate interest, skill, and background in an area that can be of value to any residency program. These experiences also make great discussion points for personal statements and interviews.

Even if you do focused specialty-specific research in a field that is not your final area of expertise, demonstrating an inclination toward academia will be a benefit and not a detriment, especially at residency programs affiliated with larger academic centers. Whatever the project, it is better to work to a tangible end rather than simply being a faceless assistant in an ongoing project. In other words, your involvement should lead to a publication, an oral abstract, or poster presentation, ideally as first author. Completing, rather than just temporarily partici-pating in, a project demonstrates organizational skills and the ability to multitask and follow through.

Finally, check the NRMP's most recent *Program Director Survey* and *Charting Outcomes in the Match* to assess the importance of research in your desired field, as well as the average number of publications by a successfully matched applicant [3, 4]. The more competitive fields have a clear proclivity for research and will be difficult to match in without a strong research background. However, do keep in mind that research experience will be less valued at community-based programs than at major academically based programs. Therefore, if you have decided that you want to train out in the community, focusing on research may not be the best way for you to spend your time.

Awards

We have already discussed the use of Alpha Omega Alpha membership as a residency program screening and ranking tool. Some programs also highly value the Gold Humanism Society. Other awards are less well known. Go to your Dean's Office and request a list of commonly given awards or scholarships. Also, search for research awards online, focusing on such pos-sibilities as postgraduate education awards (both in general and specific to medicine), research awards, leadership awards, and regional awards. If you know your future specialty, be sure to check society and conference websites for trainee awards. If applicable, check for awards geared towards advancing an underrepresented minority in medicine. Perhaps you have a talent or in-terest that sets you apart from others. You may be surprised about some of the possibilities. For instance, Tylenol offers a $10 000 scholarship to medical students as part of their Future Care Scholars Program. It may seem odd to apply to awards yourself, but in academia, you need to be your own biggest fan rather than waiting for a nomination from others.

 Insider Tip: Do not wait to be granted awards by your school or peers; research the possibilities yourself and apply. Be proactive!

Extracurricular and Extra-Extracurricular Activities

Involvement in a specialty interest group demonstrates a clear commitment to that specialty. However, the time constraints of membership versus leadership in any extracurricular club should be weighed against your study and/or research time. While a leadership position is an obvious positive feature on an application, it is a brief, possibly unnoticed line in a CV and should not be pursued at the cost of an Honors rather than High Pass grade in a course or a clinical rotation. Unless you can easily manage the obligation of club leadership, membership alone will fill the same line on a CV. Moreover, attending meetings and mixers as a member will afford you the same opportunity for making professional contacts.

"Extra-extracurricular" activities are interests and hobbies outside the scope of your education. They give a reviewer insight into your personality and make great interview conversation topics, but be careful not to cross the line from interesting to strange. Stay away from politically charged viewpoints or activities that may carry a negative connotation. Not everyone sees Cosplay or guerilla gardening as a good use of time. And while failing to mention these leisurely pursuits may feel deceptive in some way, it is important to recognize that medicine is a relatively conservative world. Your application reviewer or interviewer may be open-minded and find your penchant for extreme ironing fascinating, but more likely will consider these interests too bizarre to ignore and simply choose another applicant with the same credentials and without the "red flag."

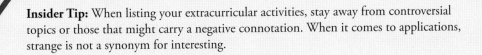

Insider Tip: When listing your extracurricular activities, stay away from controversial topics or those that might carry a negative connotation. When it comes to applications, strange is not a synonym for interesting.

In the end, we recommend reviewing the NRMP *Program Director Survey* online to see how your chosen specialty weighs USMLE scores, grades, and other features of your application [4]. Use the NRMP *Charting Outcomes in the Match* data to compare your quantitative assessments against those of applicants who successfully matched in your specialty [3]. This will help gauge your chances of making it through the initial resident applicant screening process. If your scores/grades are far from these thresholds, discuss your chances with your advisor and specialty-specific mentor. It may be time to reconsider. If you are only a little off the mark, do not fret. Focus on your positive traits, improve your secondary measures in the time that remains, bolster your application via the methods we have outlined, expand your program application list accordingly, and plan for a fourth year that will help you achieve your goals. Once you are granted an interview, you can stop second guessing your academic worth. An invitation for an interview translates into a program saying you meet their academic qualifications. Now it is time for you to shine at the interview and land that residency position.

References

1. Vidic, B. and Weitlauf, H. M. (2002) Horizontal and vertical integration of academic disciplines in the medical school curriculum. *Clinical Anatomy* **15** (3): 233–235.
2. Daley, B. J. and Torre, D. M. (2010) Concept maps in medical education: an analytical literature review. *Medical Education* **44** (5): 440–448.
3. NRMP (2011) *Charting Outcomes in the Match, 2011.* Washington, DC: National Resident Matching Program.
4. NRMP (2012) *National Resident Matching Program, Data Release and Research Committee: Results of the 2012 NRMP Program Director Survey.* Washington, DC: National Resident Matching Program.

Chapter 4

5. American Association of Colleges of Osteopathic Medical Schools Application Service (ACOMAS). Annual Osteopathic Medical School Medical School Questionnaires, 2008–09 through 2012–13 academic years; available from: http://www.aacom.org/data/graduates/Pages/default.aspx [accessed February 2014].

6. Punswick, K., *et al.* (2006) Osteopathic medical students and the allopathic licensing examination. *Journal of the International Association of Medical Science Educators* **16** (2): 93–99.

7. Hasty, R. T., *et al.* (2012) Graduating osteopathic medical students' perceptions and recommendations on the decision to take the United States Medical Licensing Examination. *Journal of the American Osteopathic Association* **112** (2): 83–89.

8. Shannon, S. (2012) Explaining the Planned Unified GME Accreditation System, in *Inside OME*. Chevy Chase, MD: American Association of Colleges of Osteopathic Medicine.

9. AOA (2013) Discussions on ACGME Unified Accreditation System, in *Inside the AOA*. Chicago, IL: American Osteopathic Association.

10. Ching, L. M. and Burke, W. J. (2011) Osteopathic distinctiveness in osteopathic predoctoral education and its effect on osteopathic graduate medical education. *Journal of the American Osteopathic Association* **111** (10): 581–584.

11. AOA Bureau of Osteopathic Medical Educators (2012) Resolution B-14. Semper D.O. AOA Approval of ACGME Residency Training. Chicago, IL: American Osteopathic Association.

12. Timeline: AOA response to ACGME changes. 2014 Last updated October 2013; available from: http://www.osteopathic.org/inside-aoa/Pages/acgme-policy-timeline.aspx [accessed February 2104].

13. ACGME (2013) *Common Program Requirements; Effective July 1, 2016*. Chicago, IL: American College of Graduate Medical Education.

14. NBOME (2014) *Information for Candidates*. Chicago, IL: National Board of Osteopathic Medical Examiners.

15. Doherty, E. M. and Nugent, E. (2011) Personality factors and medical training: a review of the literature. *Medical Education* **45** (2): 132–140.

Chapter 4

5: The Selection Process – Theirs

While the process of applying to residency is daunting, the process of recruiting and selecting future residents can be equally challenging. Selecting residents is one of the most important decisions a program can make, as they will be colleagues for at least 3 years and in some specialties up to 8 years! Most programs are looking to maximize the diversity of applicants, while assembling a cohesive residency class. Each program defines a good "fit" differently. However, in general, most programs review the submitted application for evidence of a solid work ethic and passion for learning. Positive personal attributes include good communication skills, the ability to work both independently and as a part of a team, a positive attitude, a conscientious nature, and a high energy level.

The selection process varies among programs, so that there is no uniform system for selecting residents. However, most programs divide the process into three stages:

1. Electronic Residency Application Service (ERAS®) screening/interview selection
2. Interviews
3. Ranking candidates

The ERAS program allows for an organized review of the applications. At our institution, two committee members review each application above a certain United States Medical Licensing Examination® (USMLE®) Step 1 threshold. Our Program Director reviews all applications that fall below that threshold, because we recognize that USMLE Step 1 is only one measure of future success.

Stage I	→	**Stage II**	→	**Stage III**
Interview Selection		Interviews		Ranking

Stage I: ERAS Screening/Interview Selection

ERAS breaks down each application for reviewers into nine broad categories: Summary Sheet, General Information, Couples/Visa/Other, Education, Publications, Experience, Licensure, Examinations, and Documents. One of the first sections that reviewers often look at is the summary of the applicant. There are specific components of the Summary Sheet which a program can choose to display or hide during review, such as your photograph, ethnicity, gender, or criminal background. Since the photograph is often the only visual impression of you that a program will have until interview day, it is *crucial to attach a good photograph of yourself*. You should appear well-groomed and conservatively and professionally dressed. For men, that means a suit and tie; for women, a blouse, suit jacket, or dress is most appropriate. It is definitely worth the extra money to have a professional take your picture to ensure that you are properly centered and presented in your best light. It is mind-boggling how often candidates send in a picture that is either too casual or too much like a mug shot, or do not even attach a picture at all.

Chapter 5

> **Insider Tip:** Do not underestimate the importance of attaching a great photograph of yourself in appropriate dress. This will be the only visual impression the selection committee may have of you until interview day.

Another common issue we see is a wide disparity between an applicant's appearance in the photograph and on interview day. When our review board met during a recent cycle to discuss our final applicant rank list, there was an applicant that no one recognized on the list. Attributing this to a rather unmemorable interview, he was bumped toward the bottom of the list, until one reviewer remembered the applicant who appeared clean shaven in his picture had a full beard on interview day. Even then, the remaining reviewers were dubious as to the identity of this applicant, which no doubt hurt his final ranking. Men, this is not the time to grow out your beards in support of your favorite baseball team. Women, this is not the time to indulge your curiosity about a drastic hairstyle change.

> **Insider Tip:** Do not drastically change your appearance between your submitted photograph and interview day. If you have a stellar interview early in the interview period, but looked nothing like your picture come rank time, this lack of recognition may hurt your eventual ranking.

Reviewers go through each application quickly, but pay careful attention to "red flags" such as legal misdemeanors, delayed graduation, and leaves of absence. Do not underestimate the significance of these factors nor hope that reviewers will not notice them. Address them head on by fully explaining any gaps in education, so that the program does not see this as a "red flag."

> **Insider Tip:** Do not ignore any gaps in your education. It is one of the first things a reviewer looks for in your file. Gaps in your education must be addressed in your application. Do not leave it up to the imagination of the reviewer.

A large portion of the reviewer's time is spent within the Documents section, which includes the Medical Student Performance Evaluation (MSPE), transcript, letters of recommendation (LoRs), personal statement, and board scores. The personal statement should not have any grammatical or spelling errors, because strong written communication skills are valued highly in most training programs. The 2012 National Resident Matching Program (NRMP®) *Survey of Residency Directors* revealed that the most important factors for granting interviews were USMLE Step 1 scores, LoRs, the personal statement, and grades in required clerkships, and we generally emphasize similar factors in our selection process [1]. Other important factors include the MSPE, which often includes a class ranking, and medical school reputation, as well as geography and unique personal qualities. With two reviewers analyzing an application for approximately 10 minutes each, we can spend nearly 230 hours reviewing up to 700 applications during Stage I.

> **Insider Tip:** Each application is viewed for only a few minutes, so make sure that important accomplishments are prominently highlighted in your application.

Therefore, while filling out ERAS can seem redundant when you are already attaching your curriculum vitae (CV), be sure to reiterate all your accomplishments in ERAS and fill out the form completely. Do not sell yourself short when filling out the sub-tabs by giving reviewers too much credit, expecting they will find important accomplishments in your attached CV hidden on the last page. Highlight major accomplishments at least several times so they cannot be missed even on a cursory review! The last section (Miscellaneous tab) is an excellent opportunity to highlight unique characteristics that do not fit well in the other sections. Take the time to list (and possibly briefly describe, if the title is not self-explanatory) any major awards or accomplishments, both academic and extracurricular. For example, if you were an All-American soccer player or professional violinist, make sure to list it. Accomplishments like these are not only interesting and great talking points for an interview, but also demonstrate dedication, perseverance, and the ability to multitask.

In the end, most programs assign each application a numerical score, which is an average of the evaluations of individual reviewers. The form we use at Beth Israel Deaconess Medical Center to score each applicant is shown in Figure 5.1. As you can see, this score takes into account both the strengths of the candidate and the perceived probability that an applicant will rank the program high enough to match here. Although the latter criterion is quite subjective, after participating in the match for many years, most Program Directors have a good idea of the caliber of candidate their program attracts. In addition, geography plays an important role. If you have a geographical preference because of family or friends, particularly if it is far from your current residence, emphasize this in your personal statement or in a separate email to the Program Director. For example, as an East Coast program, we tend to attract candidates with roots to the general area. We have traditionally had less success matching candidates with lifelong ties to California and Texas, and thus they represent a smaller percentage of our interviewed candidates. You may be wondering, if the mathematics of the matching algorithm dictate that all the best applicants should be placed at the top of our rank list regardless of our perceptions of whether or not they will rank us highly, why should we not interview all solid applicants in order to increase our chances of creating a class of the best applicants. However, the reality is there is a substantial cost of time and money in interviewing applicants, so we will not interview all the "great applicants" if we think it is unlikely that they will rank us highly for geographic reasons. Moreover, despite the lack of logic, there is a degree of vanity in a program's resident rank list. Programs often like to brag that they only have to go so far down

RADIOLOGY RESIDENT APPLICANT EVALUATION
BETH ISRAEL DEACONESS MEDICAL CENTER

Name:

Med. School:

INTERVIEW SELECTION GUIDELINES (0–5)

4–5	**INVITE FOR INTERVIEW (No Reservations)**
3–4	**POSSIBLY INTERVIEW (With Reservations)**
2–3	**UNLIKELY TO INTERVIEW**
1	**DO NOT INTERVIEW**

Academic Record   _____

Medical School/Clinical Experience   _____

Research Experience   _____

References (LoRs, MSPE)   _____

Potential to Contribute to Radiology   _____

Extracurricular Activities   _____

Geography   _____

OVERALL EVALUATION: (1 2 3 4 5) _____

Evaluator:_____

Figure 5.1 Sample "Radiology Resident Applicant Evaluation" form.

their rank list in order to fill all their vacant positions. As we discussed in Chapter 1: *The Match Alphabet Soup*, you should not fall victim to the same hubris.

> **Insider Tip:** If you wish to relocate as a resident, stress the reason(s) for this geographic preference in your personal statement or by email to the Program Director. In this situation, you must individualize your personal statement as you do not want to send a West Coast program a statement indicating that you have a strong desire to be in New York City. Reviewers are aware that students often apply to good programs in areas where they have no desire to live, simply as backups. Without a clear intention of the motivations to move, reviewers may not rank these applicants highly.

Based on the committee's score, applicants may be offered an interview, placed on the wait list, or declined an interview. If you are placed on the wait list, it may be of value to send an email reaffirming your specific interest in the program and reasons why you might want to train at that institution. There may be an unexpected cancellation by another applicant, opening up an interview slot for you. At our institution, in every selection cycle, up to 5% of candidates cancel interviews, so a small percentage of applicants on the wait list do eventually have the opportunity to interview. If you do need to cancel a scheduled interview, it is critical to contact the program as early as possible. Not only is this the most professional approach (you do not want to burn any bridges with an institution where you might want to do a fellowship or even join the faculty), but it also provides the program and other applicants sufficient time to fill the interview slot.

Stage II: The Interview

Interviews constitute the second stage of our selection process. The interview allows us an in-depth look at a candidate. Your role on interview day will be discussed more in depth in Chapter 10: *The Interview*. This section will briefly discuss the logistics of the process from the standpoint of Program Directors.

We begin to send our invitations approximately 2 weeks after the release of the MSPE, although some programs offer interviews prior to this. Other programs use a rolling invitation process, with invitations granted as soon as applications become available for review. Interview spots fill up *extremely* quickly, so a prompt response to the offer is strongly advised. For instance, we offer about *100 interview spots*, which fill within *1 week* following issuance of invitations.

The interview is a program's chance to get to know an applicant personally. It is also your chance to decide if this is the place where you want to train. Most programs have some idea of where each candidate would stand based upon their application alone, but the interview can substantially affect your ranking. Do not forget that the interview begins with your initial communication with the program coordinators; continues during any evening dinners or socials, interview lunches, and tours; and concludes with your formal interviews.

> **Insider Tip:** The interview extends far beyond your formal visit. Every interaction with a program is fair game, so always be on your best behavior.

The interview is a little like speed dating. It is really just a chance for an applicant and interviewer to have a quick chat and get to know each other better in order to establish whether or not you are a good fit. The interviewers are evaluating whether they can imagine working with you every day over the next few years. Interview days are long. While an applicant may interview with an average of four or five interviewers during a day, most of our interviewers will be interacting with every applicant in your group. Interviewing 100 applicants per cycle for 20 minutes each equates to more than 30 hours listening to why an applicant wants to go into that specialty or attend that program. So it is important to be upbeat and enthusiastic, even at the end of the day. Following each interview, the interviewer typically assigns a numerical score that summarizes whether he/she believes you are a good fit for the program.

Stage III: Ranking

From the program perspective, the day is not finished following the interviews. There is a wrap-up session where the interviewers and our chief residents discuss the candidates and rank them in comparison with other applicants seen that day as well as the larger interview pool. The chief residents summarize how the candidates interacted during social events, lunch, and the tour. Again, do not underestimate the importance of these interactions. We have moved candidates to the "Do Not Rank" category based upon these summaries. One of the interviewers then presents each candidate in a manner similar to the following:

> Joe Applicant is from ABC medical school. He grew up in Georgia and has been on the west coast since. He has no ties to Boston. He scored 252 on Step 1 and received a mixture of honors and high passes on his clinical rotations, including honors in medicine and a high pass in surgery. His LoRs were outstanding. He placed in the second quartile of his class. He is an avid tennis player and the Georgia state champion. I really liked him. He interviewed well, has an easy going personality, and would fit in well here. I would give him a score of 6 out of 7.

We go around the room, with all interviewers stating any points of agreement or disagreement and offering their own numerical scores. Your interviewers really are your major advocates, as they have gotten to know you the best and can make or break your candidacy. The numerical scores assigned by each interviewer are averaged and used to generate a preliminary rank list. It is rare for a candidate to be in the "Do Not Rank" category after an interview, but it is possible. Characteristics that can make a candidate "not rankable" include:

- **Inability to communicate appropriately** with the faculty, referring physicians, and fellow residents. Language barriers or extreme introversion can contribute to this perception.
- **Perception that an applicant has a highly unusual personality**, which would not fit well with the current residents.
- **A significant discrepancy within the application** that was discovered during the interview.

Shortly after the final interview session of the season, we reconvene to adjust our final rank list. By this time, reviewers are suffering from interview fatigue. Working off of the preliminary rank list generated by the interview day sessions, the Program Directors meet our full committee, which also includes our Department Chair, Vice Chair of Education, Director of Medical Student Education, faculty involved in the selection process, and chief residents.

While every program is different, we present each candidate on a PowerPoint slide with their photograph, key statistics, unique characteristics, and any important notes (likes or dislikes) that were made on interview day. For instance, comments might include "Really wants to come here. Clearly had researched our program and asked very pointed questions" or "Seemed arrogant and only interested in fringe benefits." The qualifications and personalities of the candidates are debated, sometimes hotly, and individual applicants are moved up or down based upon the group consensus. Of course, not all opinions are equal. Generally, the opinions of the Program Director, Chair, and Vice Chair of Education carry more weight. Still, the large majority of candidates will not move from their position on the preliminary rank list. Here are a few factors that may alter your rank at this stage:

- **A program receives additional information from you or a faculty member stating that you have decided that you want to train at their institution**. Many applicants send emails stating that they are ranking a program as their first choice. Program Directors know to take such letters with a grain of salt. Every year, there are such candidates who do not end up at our program despite being ranked in a position to match there. Unfortunately, this makes it more challenging if you actually do have a strong interest in one program over all the others. Sending one email reaffirming your interest in the program may be helpful. However, an email from a faculty member, either from your institution or the program's, attesting to your interest will be regarded as more reliable and thus influential.

- **There is a change in your application**. Some medical schools do not award Alpha Omega Alpha until candidates are well into the interview season. If you are fortunate enough to be awarded Alpha Omega Alpha or receive another prestigious honor, make sure to update programs about your status.

- **You become a nuisance**. Programs occasionally receive an inordinate number of emails from an applicant during the time between the interview and the rank list meeting. After completing your interviews, one email affirming interest in a program is typically sufficient. Additional emails that add important new information to your application are welcome. However, multiple emails week after week usually backfire, since programs perceive these applicants as being high maintenance, lowering them on the rank list or even classifying them as "Do Not Rank."

Reference

1. NRMP (2012) *National Resident Matching Program, Data Release and Research Committee: Results of the 2012 NRMP Program Director Survey*. Washington, DC: National Resident Matching Program.

6: Selection Process – Yours

Now that you have learned how programs select residents to interview and eventually rank, it is time to discuss how you, in turn, should select programs to which to apply. When evaluating programs, there are two main questions to keep in mind:

1. **How likely am I to be granted an interview here or be ranked in a position to match?** You need to be able to accurately gauge a program's reputation and level of competitiveness. Applying to programs far beyond your reach is a waste of time, effort, and expense.

2. **Will this program help me reach my life and career goals?** Does the program offer you the opportunities and support to help you develop your career? How happy will you be at this program? This question has different meanings to different people, and we will discuss the most popular facets to consider.

Similar to the residency program's selection process, your own selection process can be considered as consisting to three stages:

Stage I $\rightarrow$ **Stage II** $\rightarrow$ **Stage III**

Residency Application   Interviews   Ranking

However, from an organizational standpoint, it may be best to think of it as three lists:

Initial Application List $\rightarrow$ Secondary Selection Criteria List $\rightarrow$ Rank Order List (ROL)

Stage 1: Residency Application

Establishing an Application List

To begin developing an application list, you need to choose a program feature that is both crucial to you and easily searchable on the internet. For instance, if bench research is very important to you, you should apply to academic centers rather than community hospitals. Other variables such as the fabled "right fit" can only be properly assessed on interview day and should be reserved for your secondary selection criteria list. The program attributes listed below are some of the most frequently cited determining factors used by applicants when choosing a program. They are also some of the most easily assessed prior to interview day.

Geography

Geography is consistently listed as one of, if not the, top criteria that applicants use in choosing a residency program [1–4]. This reason has little to do with the program itself, but rather is related to family or friendship ties, familiarity with the area, perceived desirability of the location (e.g., safety, school system, cost of living, outside activities), job opportunities for a significant other, or the belief that their future career may be enhanced by forming contacts in that area. Multiple studies have shown that first practice locations are heavily influenced by the location of the residency training program, regardless of prior ties to the region [5–7]. If location is of the utmost importance, choose a website that allows you to sort by state. The American Medical Association (AMA)'s online database, FREIDA Online® (Fellowship and Residency Electronic Interactive Database; https://www.ama-assn.org/go/freida) includes 9500 accredited Graduate Medical Education (GME) programs that you can search by specialty, state, or training institution. You can apply for a free account online. The information listed for each program is very basic, simply the program ID number, participation in the Electronic Residency Application Services (ERAS®) or National Resident Matching Program (NRMP®), and the number of training positions offered. However, be aware that while FREIDA Online is one of the most up-to-date resources available, its accuracy is not guaranteed. Therefore, verify any information before acting on it (particularly contacting people).

Fellowship Opportunity

Come application time, most of you will know whether or not you wish to subspecialize after residency. In fact, many of you will already have a short list of subspecialty considerations. Recognizing the increased likelihood of achieving a fellowship in the same hospital as your residency program, as well as the ease of not moving just for fellowship training, many farsighted residency applicants also consider in-house fellowship opportunity when choosing a program. FREIDA Online also allows you to search for fellowship programs by the same criteria as outlined above. If you plan on pursuing a fellowship, but not necessarily at the same hospital as your residency program, remember that you will have to go through yet another application process down the road. In that case, the reputation of your residency will affect your ability to secure the fellowship of your choice.

Research

If you have set research interests or plan to practice in an academic center where research is encouraged, if not required, be sure to make this a primary focus of your search. You can generate a list by doing a geographic search and including only the large academic centers in that area, or you can generate a list by using the research award database of the National Institutes of Health (NIH) (http://report.nih.gov/award/index.cfm). In this database, you can search by location and program type (your primary interests will be "Independent Hospitals" and "Domestic Higher Education," the latter for school rather than hospital-based funding) and screen for those receiving the highest awards.

If research is of interest to you but not your primary concern, establish your list by other criteria. You can narrow it down by the NIH database results or by investigating the interests of research faculty at the programs on your list. You can usually find this information on their faculty webpage or via a PubMed (http://www.ncbi.nlm.nih.gov/pubmed) search by faculty author. Be sure to confirm the availability of research opportunity and support on interview day, as research faculty may not be involved with resident training or readily accessible. Conversations with current residents on interview day, as well as understanding how a program encourages research (such as reimbursement or allowed time for conference attendance, presence of academic mentoring programs, and research requirements for graduation), should give you good insight.

Prestige and Competitiveness

Perception of a program's prestige is a frequently cited reason for applicant interest [3, 8, 9]. Yet, of our criteria for building an application list, it can be the most confusing and stressful for medical students to assess.

Before discussing how to evaluate a program's prestige, a few cautionary notes. First, the most prestigious hospital you can rank is not always the right fit for you. If a program is too formal, cutthroat, or has an emphasis on research that is different from your own, you are unlikely to thrive there. Second, the prestige of a program is not necessarily representative of its current quality. The reputation of a program is built on the shoulders of the research, recognition, and accomplishments of their staff. Since these factors take time, it may reflect former staff. In addition, the research that contributed to a program's prestige may actually have been generated at their university affiliates and have little to do with the hospital department itself. That being said, if you are considering a role in academia or planning on pursuing a competitive fellowship, *all else being equal*, training at a prestigious residency program can benefit your career.

> **Insider Tip:** The most prestigious hospital that grants you an interview should not be automatically ranked #1 on your ROL. It may not be the right fit for you.

Given the link between university productivity and the reputation of an affiliated hospital, you will already have an idea of a program's reputation based on your college or medical school admission process. The most highly regarded schools in the country at that time are likely tied to the most prestigious hospitals and residency programs now. Your advisor and specialty specific mentors are your best resources for assessing a program's current status.

Another way to assess the prestige factor is to recognize its invariable link to a residency program's competitiveness. We can put a number on that factor – your USMLE Step 1 (or in some cases also Step 2) score. As we discussed in Chapter 5: *The Selection Process – Theirs*, residency programs realize that a USMLE score does not represent a medical student as a whole package and those not meeting this criterion will undergo an abbreviated secondary review. Be that as it may, the USMLE score cutoff of an individual program, compared with the NRMP's report of the average USMLE score of a successfully matched resident in that specialty, will give you a sense of the competitiveness of the program. Some programs post this cutoff on their websites or your advisor will have a reasonable estimate based on prior admissions. Alternatively, many residency applicants post their scores alongside interview invitations or rejections on medical student chat forums. While these can give you a rough idea of what a program is looking for, enter these sites at your own peril. Posters are under no obligation to be truthful nor is the information in any way a complete representation of their application. Use all the information available to place programs in categories, using such language as highly competitive, competitive, and less competitive. Be sure to apply to a few programs at the extremes of your own competitiveness level, which represent "reach" or "safety" programs.

While this may seem simple enough, the stress students feel when trying to account for the reputation of programs is usually born out of a desire to rank them on prestige alone and then use that list as a basis for their own ROL. Looking for answers, they turn to a broad range of published rankings, everything from *US News'* Top 100 to medical student chat rooms, only to be more frustrated when the rankings do not match. Obsessing over slight variations in these rank lists will only lead you to ignore your own career and life goals, and develop a ROL based on an assessment of the "best" programs compiled by someone else. The only utility of these lists is to employ the same categorization method as we did with USMLE score cutoffs. In other words, if a program is consistently listed in the top 25, consider it a high-quality program. There is no real difference if it is positioned 10th on one list and 15th on another.

Insider Tip: Deciding your residency program application or ROL based solely on someone else's interpretation of the "best" program is ignoring your personal goals. You may end up in a program that is not the best fit for you.

Organizing and Expanding Your Application List

According to the 2013 NRMP *Applicant Survey* [4], the successfully matched US Senior applicant submitted a median number of 29 applications (Figure 6.1). This is proportionately higher for those applying to either an advanced residency position that requires a separate Preliminary/Transitional Year of training, a backup specialty, or those high-risk applicants who are attempting to compensate with increased application numbers. Unmatched applicants submitted a median of 50 applications. The number of programs to which you should apply is an individual question based on the competitiveness of the specialty and programs to which you are applying and the merits of your application. Across all specialties, the average successful US Senior applicant interviewed at 10 programs, ranging up to 16 for Neurosurgery. Between 10 and 12 program interviews is a reasonable goal. You can review specialty-specific application and interview numbers in the 2013 NRMP *Applicant Survey* [4].

Keeping track of this many applications requires organization. The ERAS Applicant Document Tracking System (ADTS), accessible through either the top right-hand corner of the My-ERAS dashboard or at the initial sign-in page (https://www.aamc.org/students/medstudents/eras/), has greatly streamlined the application document collection and disbursement. For any given program, ADTS tracks the status of the documents and board scores you have assigned,

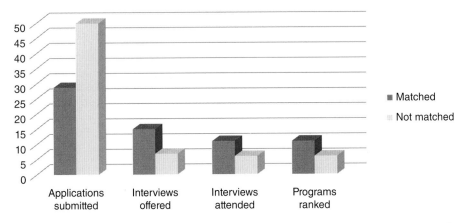

Figure 6.1 Median application data for US Seniors across all specialties in 2013. *Source*: Adapted with permission from figure 5 of [4].

including when the programs download them. Despite the efficiencies of the MyERAS system, we recommend expanding your application list into a central source spreadsheet, an application tracker, with the following information:

- Program name and Association of American Medical Colleges (AAMC) ID
- Contact information/URL
- Application document dates of upload and subsequent program download
  - ○ ERAS application
  - ○ Transcript
    - ▪ Medical school
    - ▪ United States Medical Licensing Examination® (USMLE®)/Comprehensive Osteopathic Medical Licensing Examination of the United States (COMLEX-USA®)
  - ○ Medical School Performance Evaluation (MSPE)
  - ○ Letters of recommendation
  - ○ Application requirements unique to that program, such as undergraduate or Medical College Admission Test® (MCAT®) transcript
- Invitation
  - ○ Rejected versus invited (supply the date of offer)
  - ○ Dates offered (you may need to switch later)
  - ○ Date chosen
- Competitiveness Information
  - ○ Tier assignment (high through low competitiveness)
  - ○ USMLE score cutoff
- Comments section
  - ○ Use this to record any information that led you to place a program on your list (or eventually remove it); also include any aspects of the program that you plan to investigate further at an interview

Chapter 6

> **Insider Tip:** Keep a centralized source of all your application information for easy review of status and for assessing residency program responses to your application in the various competitiveness categories.

We recommend including a comments and competitiveness ranking on your central application list, as you will be increasing or decreasing your application list as you hear back (or do not hear back) about interview dates. Many students do not have an accurate understanding of their worth and may be surprised by the response. Having this information in your central document will allow you to track the quality of programs from which you are receiving interview invitations. If your invitations are slow to come in and are mostly limited to the "competitive" or "less competitive" categories, you may be in some trouble with your current application list. Talk to your advisor and relax your criteria or geographical restraints in order to increase your application pool. Conversely, if you have received a good response from your top programs, perhaps you can free up some time and money by whittling down your safety programs or those in less desirable locations.

> **Insider Tip:** Students often misjudge their worth (usually underestimate). Be sure to have your advisor and specialty-specific mentor review your final application list. You may be surprised at which programs they suggest.

Application list organization and an updated personal calendar are crucial when it comes to scheduling interviews. Before accepting any interviews, be well versed in your school's policy for taking time off to interview. Schools generally make a distinction between time off per rotation versus the entire interview season (November through early February). Depending on the timing of your interview offers, you may need to supplement this with a vacation block. Respond promptly to interview invitations, record the offered and accepted date on your application tracker, and immediately place them in your calendar. You do not want your first contact with a residency program coordinator to be a request to change an interview date because of your scheduling error. Moreover, as the interview season progresses, programs are less likely to be able to comply with your request to switch to a different date.

Another organizational pointer is to keep an expandable folder tabbed with sections dedicated to the programs to which you are applying. The binder will serve as a depot for the incredible amount of paperwork you will receive over the next few months, which may range from medical school advisory documents to residency program interview packets (many programs do not provide a digital file so as to avoid unauthorized reproduction). You will eventually limit these sections to programs that invite you for interviews, but hold on to the information you have gathered just in case you need to reapply through the Supplemental

Offer and Acceptance Program (SOAP®). Interview packets are usually folders that include a program brochure and such supplementary material as benefits packages, information about the city (cost of living, descriptions of nearby neighborhoods, public transportation, and things to do), and childcare services. This is a large amount of material to think about at the time of the interview, and you will need to keep all of it organized for final review before submitting your ROL.

Stage 2: The Interviews

Establishing a List of Secondary Selection Criteria

Just as you created an application list when starting the application phase, you should create another as you move into the interview phase – a list of your secondary selection criteria. In order to glean the most you can from an interview, you need to have clearly established criteria of what is important for you. With these in mind, you can ask the right questions and check off the criteria that have been satisfied. The following are some of the more commonly cited secondary selection criteria, as well as some of the features you may use in assessing them:

- Quality of faculty
    - Academic accomplishment or national recognition, willingness to teach, supportive in training and later job or fellowship search, ease of interactions
    - Gender or ethnic diversity of the staff
- Quality of residents
    - Board pass rate, job or fellowship opportunities, number of publications, role in leadership positions (both in-house and in specialty organizations)
- Resident morale
    - Knowing what they know now, would they choose this program again?
    - Residents feel appreciated and supported
    - Is the program responsive to resident opinions or suggestions? Is there a system in place to address these issues?
    - Flexibility in schedule
        - Who makes the schedule? Is it often easier to arrange a short period of time off or make rotation/vacation requests of a co-resident responsible for scheduling rather than the program director or education committee?
        - If you already have or plan to have a family during residency, discretely talk to residents about the support and schedule adjustments they received
    - Do the residents socialize with each other outside of work?
- Program stability
    - Program accreditation status or prior citations
    - Recent or expected staff turnover, particularly in key positions, such as Chairman, Program Director, or any nationally recognized faculty
    - Financial stability – though rare, in this climate of healthcare reform, ask about rumors of potential program closure

- Patient population
  - May be defined by the location of the program in terms of urban versus rural
  - Within a city, population may be defined by surrounding neighborhood or partnership affiliations. For instance:
    - If a hospital has in-house drug treatment centers, nearby homeless shelters, or is partially funded to provide for free care, it will have increased exposure to certain types of pathology
    - If a hospital is in partnership with other nearby hospitals, ask if particular patients tend to be transferred to their affiliates because they have more specialized care (such as a liver or transplant center)
- Education and training requirements and opportunities
  - Formal didactics – is this protected time?
  - Typical on-the-job training experiences
  - Will there be any curricular changes in response to the proposed Accreditation Council for Graduate Medical Education (ACGME) milestones necessary for accreditation?
    - In the next accreditation cycle, the ACGME will assess a number of hospital and specialty-specific milestones. For instance, a graduation "target" for a surgical resident will be participation in "work groups or performance improvement teams designed to reduce errors and improve health outcomes" (www.acgme.org)
  - Research requirements and support
  - Number of elective weeks
    - Flexibility in choosing own elective topics
    - Opportunities for global health, business administration, quality initiatives, and other non-traditional rotations
  - Ability to interact with residents from other programs
  - Opportunities for teaching
    - Medical students (do you gain affiliation with an university?)
    - Co-residents
    - Interdisciplinary conference presentations, grand rounds.
      - These are great training experiences and excellent CV additions for those interested in academics
  - Competition with fellows for training or procedural experience
- Call schedule
  - Frequency (per training year)
  - Night float versus extended overnight shifts
  - Backup support system if exceed daily admission cap (as set by ACGME)
  - Approximately how many services/patients are you caring for at night?
  - Availability of overnight attending supervision
    - Attendings may not be located in-house while on call. If this varies from program to program, ask if there are plans to change to increased supervision.

While some prefer the safety and improved workflow associated with 24-hour in-house attending coverage, others prefer the independence to make mistakes while a trainee rather than as an attending

- ○ Call room facilities
  - ▪ If the residents are not sure where they are, you can guarantee sleep will not factor into your call shifts
- ○ Note that duty hour limitations are set by the ACGME Common Program Requirements [10]
- ○ "Duty hours must be limited to 80 hours/week, averaged over a four-week period, inclusive of all in-house call activities and all moonlighting"
  - ▪ "A Review Committee may grant exceptions for up to 10% or a maximum of 88 hours to individual programs based on a sound educational rationale"
    - – Categorically, only Neurological Surgery and Orthopedic Surgery Review Committees will grant exceptions [11]
  - ▪ "Residents must be scheduled for a minimum of one day free of duty every week [when averaged over 4 weeks]. At-home call cannot be assigned on these free days"
  - ▪ "Duty periods of PGY-1 residents must not exceed 16 hours in duration"
  - ▪ "Duty periods of PGY-2 residents and above may be scheduled to a maximum of 24 hours of continuous duty in the hospital"
- • Benefits
  - ○ Salary (relate to cost of living)
  - ○ Amount of leave (vacation, sick, maternity/paternity)
  - ○ Insurance coverage
    - ▪ Note that some programs delay coverage for a short period of time
  - ○ Discounts
    - ▪ Public transportation passes or parking (some programs offer reduced rates to trainees, others deduct these fees from your paycheck prior to income taxation)
    - ▪ Gym membership
    - ▪ Child care

Expanding and Organizing Your List of Secondary Criteria

After multiple interviews, the programs will begin to blend together, making it difficult to establish your third list – the ROL. To prepare for this final list, we recommend that you expand your selection criteria list into a spreadsheet, just as the application list was expanded into an application tracker. Maintain your selection criteria down the *y*-axis and list your interviewed programs across the *x*-axis. The NRMP recently debuted The MATCH[SM] PRISM[SM] (Program Rating and Interview Scheduling Manager) app for tracking program applications and dates of interviews granted. This links directly to the calendar on your media device – a very handy feature. It also links each interviewed program to a ranking function by listing the same selection factors assessed during the 2013 NRMP *Applicant Survey* [4] and then asks you to rate an interviewed program on each factor using one to five stars. However, we recommend that you do not use a scoring method like this to record your perceptions of an interviewed program. Instead, use your spreadsheet to record comments regarding whether a program satisfies each of your criteria. The reason for this recommendation is that the selection criteria employed by the *Applicant Survey* are vague and can be interpreted very differently. For example, you may find yourself resonating with trainees who say, "I have always learned by doing, rather than sitting in a lecture. I chose this program for the degree of autonomy a resident receives in their own education and training, as well as the lack of competition with fellows when it comes to performing procedures." Or perhaps you prefer to align yourself with the resident who notes, "The faculty here are so supportive and invested in a resident doing things right the first time. Their expertise, coupled with highly skilled fellows, means that you will learn from the best." Depending on how you define quality, you will rank these programs very differently. In addition, your priorities will evolve as you go on more interviews. Maybe the first resident's description of a quality education sounded great when you initially heard it and you gave that program five stars, but as the interview season progresses, you come to equate that style of learning with a lack of supervision. If at the end of interview season, you cannot remember why you gave a numerical rating to a program, the information is meaningless. Stick to anecdotal comments at this point. Write out important details, such as patient population or call schedule. Do not just rate the program as a "three."

Stage 3: Ranking – Preparing for Your Final ROL

Similar to how residency programs do an end-of-interview-day wrap-up and rank the day's applicants among the others they have seen thus far, you should record the details of your interview on your selection criteria list while they are fresh in your mind, preferably on the evening of your interview, and compare them against the programs you have previously visited. Consider adding a space to your spreadsheet to keep track of your preliminary ranking. Remember to rank programs based solely on your own preference, without being influenced by how likely you are to get in there. In Chapter 1: *The Match Alphabet Soup*, we discussed the matching algorithm extensively and established that attempts to "game" the Match will, if anything, have a detrimental effect on where you rank. If you need to convince yourself again, go back and review the studies. In Chapter 11: *After the Interview*, we will discuss more of the logistics of your final ROL, such as how many programs to rank and how to approach mixing specialties or advanced and preliminary programs on your primary ROL.

References

1. Aagaard, E. M., *et al.* (2005) Factors affecting medical students' selection of an internal medicine residency program. *Journal of the National Medical Association* **97** (9): 1264–1270.
2. Nuthalapaty, F. S., Jackson, J. R., and Owen, J. (2004) The influence of quality-of-life, academic, and workplace factors on residency program selection. *Academic Medicine* **79** (5): 417–425.

3. Yousuf, S. J., Kwagyan, J., and Jones, L. S. (2013) Applicants' choice of an ophthalmology residency program. *Ophthalmology* 120 (2): 423–427.

4. NRMP (2013) *Data Release and Research Committee: Results of the 2013 NRMP Applicant Survey by Preferred Specialty and Applicant Type.* Washington, DC: National Resident Matching Program.

5. Steele, M. T., *et al.* (1998) Emergency medicine resident choice of practice location. *Annals of Emergency Medicine* **31** (3): 351–357.

6. Raghavan, M., *et al.* (2012) Determinants of first practice location: among Manitoba medical graduates. *Canadian Family Physician* **58** (11): e667–e676.

7. Jarman, B. T., *et al.* (2009) Factors correlated with surgery resident choice to practice general surgery in a rural area. *Journal of Surgical Education* **66** (6): 319–324.

8. Wass, C. T., *et al.* (2003) Recruitment of house staff into anesthesiology: a re-evaluation of factors responsible for house staff selecting anesthesiology as a career and individual training program. *Journal of Clinical Anesthesia* **15** (4): 289–294.

9. Lebovits, A., Cottrell, J. E., and Capuano, C. (1993) The selection of a residency program: prospective anesthesiologists compared to others. *Anesthesia and Analgesia* **77** (2): 313–317.

10. ACGME (2013) *Common Program Requirements.* Chicago, IL: Accreditation Council for Graduate Medical Education.

11. ACGME (2011) *Frequently Asked Questions – Duty Hours. Effective 2011.* Chicago, IL: Accreditation Council for Graduate Medical Education.

Chapter 6

7: The Application

The application is a representation of your medical career to date. It includes your transcript, Medical School Performance Evaluation (MSPE), curriculum vitae (CV), United States Medical Licensing Examination® (USMLE®) or Comprehensive Osteopathic Medical Licensing Examination of the United States (COMLEX-USA®) examination scores, letters of recommendation (LoRs), personal statement, and photograph. While assembling and distributing all of this information may sound intimidating, the Association of American Medical Colleges (AAMC) has simplified the process through the creation of the Electronic Residency Application System (ERAS®) [1]. We will walk you through the logistic of ERAS, and briefly touch upon the CV and personal statement, which will be discussed in greater depth in subsequent chapters. For general reading, see the References section [2–4].

ERAS

ERAS was created in 1996 to help streamline the residency application process. Like AMCAS for medical school, ERAS is a centralized, computer-based application system managed by the AAMC, which facilitates collection, distribution, and review of your application materials. While there are other electronic match services, such as the SF Match, the vast majority of residency specialties participate in ERAS (Box 7.1).

ERAS consists of multiple components including: MyERAS, the Dean's Office Workstation (DWS), the Program Director's Workstation (PDWS), the ERAS Letter of Recommendation Portal (LoRP), and the ERAS PostOffice.

Box 7.1 Major Residency Specialties Participating in ERAS.

Anesthesia	Obstetrics and Gynecology
Dermatology	Orthopedic Surgery
Diagnostic Radiology	Otolaryngology
Emergency Medicine	Pathology
Family Medicine	Pediatrics
General Surgery	Physical Medicine and Rehabilitation
Internal Medicine	Plastic Surgery
Neurological Surgery	Psychiatry
Neurology	Radiation Oncology
Nuclear Medicine	Transitional/Preliminary

You will use MyERAS throughout the application process. Through MyERAS, you enter contact information; generate a CV-like application detailing your educational, research, and extracurricular pursuits; create and edit your personal statement; authorize release of your USMLE or COMLEX examination transcripts; identify your letter writers and track the progress of LoR submissions; and choose the programs to which you want to submit your application. Your Dean's Office, the National Board of Medical Examiners (NBME), and your letter writers are all able to directly submit necessary support documents such as the MSPE to ERAS at the appropriate time, so that your programs of interest are able to download your application for review.

ERAS Token and Registration

The ERAS season for the 2015 Match begins in April (July for International Medical Graduates (IMG)), when your Dean's Office (or Educational Commission for Foreign Medical Graduates (ECFMG®) for IMGs) will generate a unique alphanumeric token that will allow you to register. An updated users guide is also released highlighting changes in the interface and providing instructions for generating and submitting your application. It is important to register for ERAS early (even if you are not quite ready to fill out your application), because it allows your Dean's Office to begin entering your documentation. While you cannot submit your application until September 15, you will need much of this time to review and refine your application and support materials. Should you be applying for a field that uses an alternative program to ERAS – such as Urology, which conducts the Urology Residency Match Program through the American Urological Association (AUA; www.auanet.org) or Ophthalmology or Neurotology, which use the SF Match (www.sfmatch.org) – make sure to visit the appropriate website and register early.

✓ **Insider Tip:** Register and begin filling in your application early!

When you register, you will be able to complete your ERAS profile. Among other material, this includes your email, mailing, and telephone contact information, which is crucial both to allow ERAS to reach you concerning problems related to your application and so that programs can contact you to arrange for interviews. Make sure that the email address you list for the application is one you check regularly and a professional one (more on this in Chapter 8: *The Curriculum Vitae*). Include either your cellular or the home phone number of the place you will be living during the application season (i.e., not your parents' phone number). If you have a smartphone (and at this point, only a few of our older attendings do not), then it is essential to have your email synched to it, as many interview invitations are delivered by email and the choice dates fill quickly.

You can now begin working on your ERAS application. The ERAS program site is actually quite user friendly. It consists of four major tabs: Dashboard, Application, Documents, and

Programs. The Dashboard tab provides you with an overview to monitor the progress of your application, determine whether LoRs have been completed and assigned to programs, and see a list of the programs to which you have applied. The rest of this chapter will focus on the three remaining tabs – Application, Documents, and Programs.

MyERAS Application Tab

The CV (curriculum vitae = Latin for "course of (one's) life") is literally a bullet-point listing of your career activities and achievements. Hopefully, you have an existing CV that has been updated throughout medical school (see Chapter 8: *The Curriculum Vitae*, for further information about creating a CV). Under the Application section of MyERAS, you will input your CV into the program. MyERAS contains separate sections for:

- General Information
- Education: Undergraduate and graduate
- Medical School Education
- Training
- Experience: Work, volunteer, and research
- Publications
- Licensure Information
- Medical Licenses
- Self Identification
- Language Fluency
- Miscellaneous

Each individual subsection can be saved separately and all the material can be viewed in either CV or ERAS format. There are two things to consider for all of these subsections. First, always be completely honest in your activities and accomplishments. Particularly in the digital age, it is very easy to fact-check and discover any embellishments, which many programs would consider sufficient to summarily reject your application. Remember that specialists in academic medicine frequently know each other well, so it is dangerous to list a research or clinical mentor if you did not actually work with that individual or to overstate your participation in a given project. Second, everything you write in your application is fair game for the interview. If you mention a research project on *in vitro* analysis of cardiac myocytes, then be prepared to talk about the topic to some degree, even if you participated in the project 10 years ago. This also applies to language and hobbies. Applicants indicating that they are fluent in French or Spanish have been asked questions in these languages, and applicants have even been asked to sing or do origami if they are included as hobbies.

Insider Tip: Be honest! Embellishments can easily be identified!

Chapter 7

Match Timeline	
Spring	Complete subinternship/advanced elective in the specialty to which you will be applying and be on the lookout for attendings to write LoRs
	Plan your fourth-year schedule to include away electives, as well as vacation or easy electives during the interview period
	Review the MyERAS user guide
	Obtain token for accessing ERAS from the Dean's Office
	Register for ERAS and begin working on your application; you can select your programs of interest, but your application materials will not yet be transmitted to them
	Obtain a professionally taken photograph
June	Continue working on your personal statement and CV
	Determine school policy for MSPE
July	IMG applicants can register for ERAS; access token through ECFMG
August	Complete your personal statement and CV, and ensure that LoRs are completed
	Review transcript and MSPE
September 15	Begin applying to Accreditation Council for Graduate Medical Education (ACGME)–accredited programs; in turn, they can download and view your application and support materials (except the MSPE)
	Register for the National Resident Matching Program (NRMP®); do so before November 30 to avoid a late fee
October 1	MSPEs are released to programs
Mid/late October to early February	Interviews! Each specialty is different in both the timing of invitations and the actual dates for interviews
February	NRMP rank order lists (ROLs) are certified in late February
Mid March	Match Week!
	SOAP starts Match Week

Make sure to consult the AUA and SF Match websites for their deadlines, if applicable. Check www.aamc.org/students/medstudents/eras for current deadlines.

MyERAS Documents Tab

The documents section allows you to list the authors of your LoRs, submit your personal statement, and authorize release of your USMLE transcripts. Foreign graduates have additional requirements (see Chapter 13: *International Medical Graduate Specifics*).

LoRs

The LoR adds additional perspective about your performance, beyond your grades, application, and MSPE. The vast majority of letters speak glowingly about the candidate, so anything less can be a "red flag." Good letters are those that comment in detail about your performance, work ethic, and personal traits.

In a perfect world, you are golfing buddies with the Chairman of your department, who is prepared to write an effusive letter highlighting your accomplishments, performance in clinical activities, and the scholarly work you performed together. Chairmen and then Program Director letters tend to carry the most weight, as they are often widely recognized names in the field. After these individuals, senior faculty with administrative responsibilities and medical clerkship directors are the next most desirable. Letters from junior faculty carry less weight. If asking for letters from an instructor or assistant professor, make sure you know that they will be spectacular (to counteract their low academic ranking). Never ask a resident or fellow to write one of your primary letters.

> **Insider Tip:** The letters that carry the most weight are from senior members of the field.

The difficult balance that you have to strike is making sure that the people you ask are prepared to write excellent letters. As long as you have performed reasonably well with them in the lab or on the wards, most of those you ask will agree to write a LoR. But that does not guarantee they will write a great letter. You may prefer slightly more junior faculty members who know you well, if you believe they will write stronger letters than a more senior person who has only rounded with you once or twice. It is particularly helpful to have letter writers who have worked closely with you, either in direct interaction during a clerkship or as collaborators in a research project. Similarly, if your CV indicates that you have worked closely with a particular person on a research project, it will be strange if there is no letter from that individual.

> **Insider Tip:** In the end, it is most important to get a great LoR from someone who knows you well.

Always be on the lookout for opportunities to obtain excellent LoRs. Obviously, doing research with someone is a good way to become familiar with a faculty member. Alternatively, if you worked on a particularly challenging or rewarding clinical case, distinguished yourself in the care of a particular patient, or developed a good rapport with a faculty member on a clinical rotation, keep that person in mind as a possible letter writer and jot down the circumstances behind your relationship. The best time to ask for a letter is a short time after you have received a favorable evaluation from an attending on the rotation. It is important to ask for the letter soon after the rotation, as faculty members may be flooded with requests as the application deadline nears and their memory of your performance may have faded. Before deciding on a potential letter writer, make sure that you have received your clinical evaluation on the rotation, as you do not want someone who has given you unfavorable marks writing your LoR.

When asking for a letter, make sure to present yourself in a professional manner. If you do not interact frequently and casually with your letter writer, it is best to ask for an appointment. Dress appropriately and have a printed CV. During you interaction, try to gently refresh their memory of the highlights of your work together. Always give letter writers a graceful way to refuse, particularly if they seem somewhat disinterested. Since you are looking for a stellar letter, it is reasonable to phrase your request something like the following: "I was wondering whether

Chapter 7

you would be able to write me a strong letter of recommendation." If there is a lukewarm response, it is probably best to keep searching for someone else.

Within ERAS, you generate a Letter Request Form that is specific to each writer. First, you must enter the name, title, and department of the writer. This will be printed on the form with your name, contact information, AAMC ID, ERAS letter ID, and specialty. While you can assign the letter writer to one or more specialties, this information is not seen by the programs. You give the forms to all letter writers, who can either have the letter uploaded by your Dean's Office (by following instructions on the form) or upload it themselves if they register for the ERAS LoR portal. In theory, if your Dean's Office receives the letter, staff in that office can unofficially assess how complimentary it is. This can aid you in deciding which letters to ultimately send out.

The form also has an option for you to waive the right to see your letter. Programs strongly prefer that you do this, rightfully believing that this will result in letter writers being more open and honest if they know that you are not going to read what they write. Therefore, we believe there is little benefit, and potentially harm, if you do not waive your rights to see the recommendation. You have already put in hard work to make sure that you have secured the best possible letters, and the selection committee may discount your letters should you not waive your right to see them.

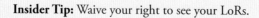

Insider Tip: Waive your right to see your LoRs.

The ERAS site allows applicants to submit four LoRs, but make sure you check the website of each program to which you are applying for specific requirements. For example, the General Surgery site at the University of California at San Francisco (http://www.surgery.ucsf.edu/education–training/academic-programs/general-surgery-residency-program/how-to-apply.aspx) asks for three LoRs, including one Chairman letter "if possible." It is generally suggested that you not submit any additional LoRs unless you are certain that it will aid your application, such as a letter from a senior member of the department to which you are applying. Extra letters beyond the number requested add potential uncertainty to your application and increase the workload of your evaluators.

Insider Tip: Make sure you know each program's specific requirements.

While you are allowed to submit only a certain number of letters to each program, you are permitted to request additional letters that can be saved within ERAS. Some applicants may ask for LoRs from multiple people. In this way, you can select which letters to send to specific programs. As most applicants waive their rights to view their LoRs, you could unknowingly receive one that is lukewarm. By sending a different combination of letters to various programs, you can limit the damage a poor letter could cause.

Insider Tip: Consider sending different letters to different institutions to minimize the impact of an unfavorable letter.

Make sure to send a note or email of thanks after receiving your letter. Your letter writers will appreciate it and you may need them to make calls on your behalf later in the application process!

Insider Tip: Make sure to thank your letter writers.

Personal Statement

The personal statement is your chance to make your application more than just a list of grades, test scores, and activities. You have complete control of the message conveyed to the programs and interview committees, and can include insights about your interest and enthusiasm for the specialty, skills and experiences, and future goals and motivations. As you are starting with a completely blank piece of paper, this process naturally can be unnerving and frustrating. It probably has also been a while since you have written an "essay" or anything other than History and Physical Examinations (H&Ps), Subjective, Objective, Assessment, and Plan (SOAP) notes, and the occasional scientific manuscript. There are numerous possible approaches, but the bottom line is to find a theme that can relate the real you, your career choice, and future goals to your audience.

It is important to start the process early, at or near the beginning of the summer and as soon as you know the specialty to which you want to apply. Feed off the inspiration that led to this decision. Write and rewrite your personal statement several times before showing it to anyone else for comments and suggestions. Do not get frustrated if you start on a blank sheet of paper or computer screen more than once, for this is a *very* common occurrence. Ultimately, you will craft a great statement that expresses to the selection committee the precise message you want to convey.

As you are likely to draft your personal statement in a program such as MS Word, there are a few things to consider. First, proofread everything yourself in addition to using spell-check. Especially in the world of autocorrect, you want to do both to avoid a similar, but incorrect, word automatically substituted for your intended word. Also, make sure to send everything to someone else for review, since a fresh set of eyes is always valuable. Programs that offer the ability to "track changes" are valuable to manage the suggestions of your editors. These should not all be immediately adopted, instead carefully scrutinized to make sure they do not drastically alter your tone or the meaning you want to convey. Second, the ERAS programming may not be perfectly compatible with the formatting used in Word. Therefore, it is a good idea to copy the text into a plain-text editor such as Notepad, which removes all the formatting before you paste it into ERAS. In this way you can reread all the information within ERAS to make sure

Chapter 7

that everything transferred appropriately. Specifically, review all punctuation (such as exclamation (!), question (?), and quotation ("…") marks) to make sure they were not inadvertently converted into extraneous symbols.

For a detailed discussion of the personal statement, see Chapter 9: *The Personal Statement*.

USMLE/COMLEX Transcripts

You need to have your USMLE ID in order to authorize the release your transcripts (and your National Board of Osteopathic Medical Examiners (NBOME) ID for your COMLEX transcripts) and designate the specific programs that should receive them. The National Board of Medical Examiners (NBME) (for US medical graduates) and ECFMG (for IMGs) charge a one-time fee ($70 for ERAS 2014; a separate $70 is required for COMLEX) to send your transcripts. This fee is the same regardless of the number of programs to which you apply and is included in your invoice when you apply to programs. Remember that all scores on the transcript at the time of transmission are sent, so that you cannot pick and choose which ones to include. Nevertheless, you can retransmit your scores if you subsequently take USMLE Step 2. It is your responsibility to know the various requirements of specific programs and states regarding completion of USMLE Step 2.

MSPE

The MSPE (the former "Dean's letter"), which is not transmitted until October 1, is handled directly by your Dean's Office. The MSPE was rated as the eighth most important factor in selecting whom to interview according to the 2012 NRMP *Program Director Survey*. Unfortunately, applicants have limited influence over what is written in their MSPE, because it is based upon medical school performance and accomplishments. Program Directors pay particular attention to the last paragraph, which often categorizes students into class percentiles. Some medical schools, including some that are highly ranked, do not stratify students, making interpretation of the MSPE more difficult. While you have little say over your ranking, you do have some influence over the composition of your letter. Medical schools often require copies of your CV and personal statement before writing the MSPE. Deans often highlight the activities and accomplishments that you emphasize in these documents. Consequently, if you want them to stress that you have completed a notable research project or are an accomplished musician, highlight these facts prominently in the CV you give them.

Your MSPE includes grades received during each rotation and excerpts from your preceptors. Make sure to review your medical school transcript to make sure there are no errors. Depending on the school, you may be involved in drafting or reviewing portions of the letter itself, and most will at least let you view the final version. Carefully review the transcript for accuracy, for you do not want it to appear that you received a HP (High Pass) instead of an H (Honors) because of sloppy transcription.

Photograph

While listed as optional, it is advisable to include a photo of yourself to help the committee better remember you during the ranking conversations. Some programs also have the option of viewing photographs during the interview selection process. With so many applicants, especially for larger Medicine and Pediatrics programs, this is just another way to be remembered. However, you do not want to be remembered for the wrong reason. Take a photo specifically for the purpose of your application; do not just crop yourself out of a previous picture. Consider hiring a professional photographer if you do not have a friend or family member who can take a good photograph of you. A standard photograph should be 2.5 × 3.5 inches, or at most 3 × 4 inches. Dress in professional attire and stand in front of a neutral background. Men should be dressed in a suit, tie, and dress shirt. Women should be dressed as they would for interviews. Most importantly, comb/brush your hair and *smile*! You would be surprised how many submitted photos look like mug shots. A picture is the only visual image members of the selection committee will have of you after the memory of the interview fades from their minds.

MyERAS Programs Tab

Assigning Programs

You can search for and select programs to which you wish to apply at any time before September 15, when applications are sent out. These will appear in the "Programs Selected" tab. Before you pay your invoice and submit your application, you can add and remove programs at will. You can then assign documents to each program in this list. In theory, you can send a specific personal statement to each program, or each type of program if you are applying to more than one program (such as preliminary and advanced), though this is by no means necessary or recommended. If you choose to do this, remember not to accidentally send the personal statement intended for program X to program Y. You cannot assign a LoR until you have finalized the author and it is available in the ERAS PostOffice. As with the personal statements, you can send specific letters to specific programs. Remember that you need to know the requirements of the programs to which you are applying with respect to LoRs and exam scores. Some programs require USMLE Step 2 and others ask for four letters (one from a specific member of the faculty, such as the Chairman).

You can use the Apply to Programs section to apply to your list of programs (once you have certified your application) *or* to preview your invoice and the "Assignments Report" to review which program is receiving which documents. Remember, it is a flat $95 for the first 10 programs to which you apply under the same specialty for ERAS 2015, and an additional $10 each for programs 11–20, $16 each for programs 21–30, and $26 each for programs 31 and above (all fees non-refundable). If you choose to submit additional applications after your initial applications were sent in September, it is your responsibility to ensure that these programs are still accepting applications. If ERAS has been notified by the program that they are closed to additional applications, you will not be permitted to submit one.

Submitting Your Application

Having completed and thoroughly edited each of the sections, you are ready to certify and submit the application. Once you submit the application, it can no longer be edited. Therefore,

Chapter 7

be absolutely sure that the application is ready to go. There is no built-in spelling or grammar check, so double or triple check for both. Before certifying, you can generate a preview of the application in the exact "application" and "CV" forms that will be received by the programs. Use these opportunities to make sure that there are no errors and that everything looks exactly as you want it.

> **Insider Tip:** Submit your application on September 15 or as soon as possible thereafter!

You really want to send your application in as soon as you can, so do not wait for a change in status of a project or award, which you can always communicate directly to your programs of interest. You must certify that you have read the policies of ERAS and AAMC before finally submitting your application, which then will be sent to programs on your list.

Once you submit your application, apply to specific programs (on or after September 15) and pay your invoice. Your documents will be immediately transmitted, except for the MSPE, which is only available on October 1.

Keep an open line of communication with your programs of interest, especially if you have any key updates to your application. Otherwise, wait patiently for your interview invitations to arrive, be kind to the program administrative staff when arranging your interviews, and good luck!

References

1. Electronic Residency Application Service (ERAS®) for Applicants; available from: https://www.aamc.org/students/medstudents/eras/ [accessed June 2014].
2. Katta, R. and Samir, D. (2009) *The Successful Match: 200 Rules to Succeed in the Residency Match.* Houston, TX: MD2B.
3. Le, T., Bhushan, V., and Shenvi, C. (2010) *First Aid for the Match*, 5th edn. New York, NY: McGraw-Hill Medical.
4. Smith, R. P. (2000) *From Medical School to Residency: How to Compete Successfully in the Residency Match Program.* New York, NY: Springer.

8: The Curriculum Vitae

The curriculum vitae (CV) is a summary of your professional and academic activities and accomplishments. You may be more familiar with writing a résumé, which is similar in that it provides a list of your training and qualifications. However, a CV is utilized in the academic world because it provides a reviewer, such as a member of a Resident Selection Committee, with a succinct yet comprehensive view of your skills, academic achievements, and interests. Unlike a résumé, which is generally limited to one or two pages, a CV can be several pages long and grows with your academic productivity. As academics are generally involved in multiple projects, have clinical responsibilities, or have publications and presentations in multiple stages of review, a CV should be considered as a dynamic document that will be updated constantly throughout your career. Ideally, you have maintained a CV throughout medical school. Otherwise you may have to create one *de novo* by racking your memory for awards or raiding your computer for saved presentations. Either way, you must prepare or update a formal CV for residency application. First, it will simplify your Electronic Residency Application Service (ERAS®) application, since you can input your CV material directly into MyERAS application subsections. Second, you will submit copies of your CV to the Dean for your Medical Student Performance Evaluation (MSPE) and to those who will be writing your letters of recommendation (LoRs). It is also useful to bring a copy of your CV to interviews, just in case your application folder is not readily available. While the CVs of seasoned faculty members may be several pages, those of residency applicants are typically only one to three pages in length. After the Name and Contact Information and Education sections, you can arrange your CV in whichever order highlights your most significant accomplishments. If you have a strong research background and publications, lead with this. If you have won several awards, then those should be featured up front. The information in the middle and bottom of the CV is often overlooked, so it is critical to prioritize the most important sections by placing them first. For general reading, see the References section [1–6].

> **Insider Tip:** While the CV of an academic attending is often many pages long, do not substitute quality for quantity in an attempt to reach that goal. The CV of a typical resident applicant is shorter ranging from one to three pages in length.

Standard Elements of a CV

While there are variations on the format and layout of a CV, Box 8.1 outlines the basic components.

> **Box 8.1** Standard Elements of a CV.
>
> Name and Contact Information
> Education
> Work and Research Experience
> Publications
> Awards
> Professional Memberships
> Extracurricular Activities
> Personal Information/Interests

Despite the simplicity of this structure, there are ways to both highlight and diminish your achievements. Take the sample CV shown in Figure 8.1, which seems straightforward and satisfies the basic elements. However, there are certainly ways to improve it. We will use this failed opportunity as a discussion point for the "dos and don'ts" of CV writing.

Name and Contact Information

Use the same name that appears on your ERAS profile. Boldface your name and set it at a larger font size than the remainder of your CV. Do not include your social security number. As with your ERAS profile, the phone number and address that you use should be the one at which you can easily be reached. Do not use the phone number of your parents, unless that is the home where you will be staying. It is unusual for a program to call you directly, but be prepared for this rare scenario and present yourself in the best light possible. Check your voicemail message greeting before the start of the interview season. Make sure it is a professional message such as:

> Hello, this is Jim Fleischner. I'm sorry to have missed your call. Please leave your name, number, and message, and I will call you back as soon as possible.

Obtain a proper email account. Do not use informal email addresses such as "drpacs", "er_doc", or in the case of the sample CV "gas_man." An example of an appropriate email to include would have been, *FirstName_LastName2004@gmail.com.*

> **Insider Tip:** Retain formality in your CV and in all your dealings with residency programs.

Education

List your medical school and any undergraduate training including post-baccalaureate. Include, location, degrees earned, areas of study, and month/year of enrollment and date of

Jim A. Fleischner

Present Mailing Address
8 Baron Court
Hanover, MA 01810
Preferred Phone: 555-267-1451
gas_man@gmail.com

Permanent Mailing Address
99 Gardner Court
Brookline, MA 02897
Alternate Phone: 555-267-6009

Education

University of Pennsylvania Medical School, Philadelphia, PA, **M.D.**	2000-2004
Undergraduate - Brown University, Providence, RI B.S. with Honors in Biochemistry *Magna cum Laude*	1995-1999

Work Experience & Research Experience:

UPenn Emergency Medicine Department, Philadelphia, PA — 2002-2004
Lab Assistant, Dr. Todd Hollander
Assistant with collection and analysis of data in patients undergoing emergency room physician-performed ultrasound of the gallbladder

National Cancer Institute, Bethesda, MD — 1999-2000
Lab Assistant, Dr Mark Blumberg
Assisted with western blots, PCR, and Elisa assays to help characterize protein kinase C.
Assisted with data collection and manuscript preparation.

Brown University, Providence, RI — 1998-1999
ER Reading Room Clerk, Samuel Arroyo, MD
Answered telephone calls and recorded information regarding requested exams for the resident and attending radiologist to review.

Publications

Peer Reviewed Journal Articles/Abstracts

Lorenzo AS, **Fleischner J,** Bottorff DA, Garfield SH, Stone JC, Blumberg M. Phorbol Esters Modulate the Ras Exchange Factor RasGRP3. *Cancer Res.* 2002; 55:938-949.

Pak Y, Smith IJ, Varady J, **Fleischner J**, Lorenzo AS, Blumberg M, and Wang S. Structural Basis of High Affinity Ligands to Protein Kinase C: Prediction of the Binding Modes Through a New Molecular Dynamics Method and Evaluation by Site Directed Mutagenesis. *J Med Chem.* 2001; 44:1690-1701.

Poster Presentation

Fleischner J, Hollander T. Discrepancy rate between emergency department physician and radiologist performed ultrasound in the evaluation of acute cholecystitis. University of Pennsylvania Research Day. June 2003.

Awards

Twenty First Century Scholars Award University of Pennsylvania	2000
Pre-IRTA Fellowship National Cancer Institute	1999

Membership and Honorary/Professional Societies

American Medical Association
Massachusetts Medical Society
American Academy of Emergency Medicine

Extracurricular Activities

University of Pennsylvania School of Medicine Student Medical Clinic	2001 – 2004
Brown University Homeless Shelter	1998 - 1999

Helped feed homeless people in the Rhode Island region.

Hobbies & Interests

Skiing, tennis, basketball

Figure 8.1 CV Sample 1: a missed opportunity (see Figure 8.2 for an enhanced version of this CV).

Chapter 8

graduation (or expected graduation). Do not include your high school. If you graduated with distinction, such as *summa cum laude,* or received other honors at graduation, mention them at this point. Consider including your GPA (grade point average) if it was stellar, but otherwise it should be omitted. Some candidates include a separate section for United States Medical Licensing Examination® (USMLE®) scores. If your USMLE scores are truly outstanding (greater than 250), consider including them on your CV. If you are a foreign medical graduate, you should include a separate Licensure and Certification section, which lists both your USMLE scores as well as your Educational Commission for Foreign Medical Graduates (ECFMG®) certification.

Work and Research Experience

This section should not be a repository for every project or job in which you have participated. Instead, list work, research, and volunteer experiences relevant to medicine, including work done in research laboratories and companies. Generally, your summer job waiting tables as a high school student should be excluded, unless there is a specific and significant reason to include them. As in the remainder of the CV, experiences should be listed in reverse chronological order, with the most recent experience first. List your role, Principal Investigator, institution (including city and state), and dates of participation. Later you can detail your role in the project and relevant project outcome(s) using bullet-point phrases. These should be concise descriptions using action verbs that explain your duties and accomplishments. Avoid using the same verb twice on your CV, or at least in the same listing. A simple online search of action verbs will produce a multitude of choices. The writer of our sample CV fell victim to this mistake, using the verb, "assisted" numerous times and in one instance even accidentally replacing it with the noun, "assistant." The edited version of our sample (Figure 8.2) uses power verbs and enhanced descriptions of his activities, accentuating the importance of his role.

Insider Tip: Word your descriptions to highlight your accomplishments. Avoid passive language, instead using *action verbs* to clearly indicate the skills you have gained.

Publications

Include abstracts, papers, and presentations in which you were an author, even if not the first. Boldface your name in the citation to help the reader find your position on the author line. Papers characterized as "in press" are interpreted as accepted and carry far more weight than those listed as "submitted," which have not yet been accepted. Nevertheless, both should be included in your CV.

Awards

List awards and scholarships that you have won in medical school and as an undergraduate. Include a line explaining the significance of the award, unless it is well-known in medical circles

Jim A. Fleischner

Present Mailing Address	Permanent Mailing Address
8 Baron Court	99 Gardner Court
Hanover, MA 01810	Brookline, MA 02897
Preferred Phone: 555-267-1451	
Jim_Fleischner2004@gmail.com	

Education

University of Pennsylvania Medical School, Philadelphia, PA	2000-2004
M.D.	
Undergraduate - Brown University, Providence, RI	1995-1999
B.S. with Honors in Biochemistry, *Magna cum Laude*	

Work Experience and Research Experience

UPenn Emergency Medicine Department, Philadelphia, PA   2002-2004
Lab Assistant, Dr. Todd Hollander
Responsible for collection and analysis of data regarding emergency room physician-performed gallbladder ultrasound in order to assess prevalence, accuracy, work-flow impact, and reimbursement issues.

National Cancer Institute, Bethesda, MD   1999-2000
Lab Assistant, Dr. Mark Blumberg
Performed western blots, polymerase chain reaction (PCR), and Elisa assays, data analysis, and participated in manuscript preparation validating protein kinase C as a potential therapeutic target for cancer in mouse models.

Brown University, Providence, RI   1998-1999
ER Reading Room Clerk, Dr. Samuel Arroyo
Acted as a liaison between referring physicians and attending radiologists by collecting preliminary reports and consultation requests, patient information, and coordinating responses.

Publications

Peer Reviewed Journal Articles/Abstracts
Lorenzo AS, **Fleischner J**, Bottorff DA, Garfield SH, Stone JC, Blumberg M. Phorbol Esters Modulate the Ras Exchange Factor RasGRP3. *Cancer Res.* 2002; 55:938-949.

Pak Y, Smith IJ, Varady J, **Fleischner J**, Lorenzo AS, Blumberg M, and Wang S. Structural Basis of High Affinity Ligands to Protein Kinase C: Prediction of the Binding Modes Through a New Molecular Dynamics Method and Evaluation by Site Directed Mutagenesis. *J Med Chem.* 2001; 44:1690-1701.

Poster Presentation
Fleischner J, Hollander T. Discrepancy rate between emergency department physician and radiologist performed ultrasound in the evaluation of acute cholecystitis. University of Pennsylvania Research Day. June 2003.

Awards

Twenty First Century Scholars Award University of Pennsylvania   2000
    Full tuition scholarship based upon outstanding academic achievement, demonstrated leadership, and
    unique life experiences.
Pre-IRTA (Intramural Research Training Award) Fellowship National Cancer Institute   1999
    Research fellowship based upon academic potential as a leader in the field of oncology.

Membership and Honorary/Professional Societies

American Medical Association
Massachusetts Medical Society
American Academy of Emergency Medicine

Extracurricular Activities

University of Pennsylvania School of Medicine Student Medical Clinic	2001-2004
Brown University Homeless Shelter	1998-1999

Hobbies and Interests

Skiing, tennis, basketball

Figure 8.2 CV Sample 2: an edited version of our first sample CV (changes highlighted in blue).

Chapter 8

(such as being named Alpha Omega Alpha or Phi Beta Kappa). For instance, in our sample CV, Jim Fleischner has won the Twenty First Century Award from the University of Pennsylvania, a little known but prestigious award. The expanded description in our edited version is much more impressive to the reader.

Insider Tip: Explain the significance of lesser-known awards.

Professional Memberships

List professional societies to which you belong. Since they are usually free or of little cost to join as a student member, there is everything to be gained from becoming a member of these societies. If you have participated in a committee or leadership position, highlight that either within this section or with your other medical student organization positions in the extracurricular activities section.

Extracurricular Activities

Here you can include those activities that do not qualify as work, volunteer, or research experience. The same principles apply: include only relevant activities, provide a short "blurb" in bullet form to highlight what you did for the group, and use action words.

Personal Information/Interests

This is typically the last line of the CV and should list hobbies, interests, and special skills, such as language proficiency. While only one or two lines, be aware that this is probably one of the sections most closely scrutinized by interviewers. Interviewers are desperate for things to get/keep the conversation flowing, and hobbies are always a good topic for discussion. As mentioned, anything in this and the remainder of the application is fair game, so do not overstate your abilities – someone may call your bluff!

Other Common CV Insider Tips

- **Do not make a grammatical error, especially if you are a foreign medical graduate.** Edit your CV *multiple* times, and have close friends and family do so as well. Make sure to check spelling and grammar using Microsoft Word or whatever word processing program you are using. If you are a foreign medical graduate and have grammatical errors, it is doubtful that you will be granted an interview no matter how strong a candidate you are.
- **Be consistent with the layout/formatting of the various entries within each of the sections.** For example, in our sample CV in Figure 8.1 there are different uses of single/double spaces after full stops, different uses of '&' and 'and' in section

headings, inconsistent use of 'hyphens' in number ranges for years, different spacing above/below section headings, varied use of colons at the end of section headings, an extraneous comma after 'PA' in first 'Education' entry, varied use of full stops in the 'M.D.' qualification and 'Dr.' abbreviations, etc. These inconsistencies have been correct in the edited version in Figure 8.2.

- **Ensure that your CV appears professional.** Print your CV using a laser printer and use CV quality 8.5 × 11-inch bond paper. Your margins should be set at 1 inch on all sides so that it does not appear too crowded.
- **Do not exaggerate your accomplishments.** It is very easy for Program Directors to go on the web to check the accuracy of your publications and awards. Do not falsely represent yourself. In one recent study investigating misrepresentation of research qualifications by radiology residents [7], there was a misrepresentation rate of 1.9% among US graduates and 8.8% among foreign medical graduates.
- **Do not make your sentences too complicated.** Keep your sentences tight and professional. For example, this sentence is a bit wordy:

> Performed western blots to isolate sonic hedgehog protein, which helped elucidate its role in the protein C kinase pathway.

It could easily be broken into two separate sentences as follows:

> Isolated sonic hedgehog protein using western blots. Investigated the role of sonic hedgehog in the protein C kinase pathway.

- **Do not use first person pronouns.** Avoid using the words "I" and "we" in your CV. Also, do not use third-person pronouns to refer to yourself, such as "he" or "she."
- **Do not use abbreviations that are not universally recognized.** Only use abbreviations that are widely known, such as USA (United States of America). If an abbreviation is obscure, include the proper title.

Figure 8.3 gives another example of a well-organized CV with accompanying comments.

General comments

This CV is well formatted with a consistent layout and uses a standard font (e.g., Times New Roman) in 11 or 12 point size. You should use one or at most two font styles throughout the CV. This example also uses an Arial font and boldfacing, as well as solid lines to divide individual sections. The dates are separated from the accomplishments and are listed on the left-hand side of the page. Notice that since the CV contains two pages, the candidate has included his name and the page number at the top of page 2, in case the pages become separated. He employs bullet points to highlight his role in activities or help clarify awards or positions. Underlining items or capitalizing all letters in a word on a CV is strongly discouraged.

While the education section should always be listed first in a CV, the sections that follow it should be arranged in a strategic way to highlight an applicant's strengths. Candidate Sam Jones has a very impressive list of awards and extracurricular activities, including membership

Sam E. Jones

Permanent Address
31 Flectcher Ave
Ogden, UT 84001

School Address
73 Parkman Street
Brookline, MA 02446
samjones@hotmail.com
(555) 645-2163

Education

2010–present **Boston University School of Medicine**, Boston, MA
MD expected July 2014

2006–2010 **Emory University**, Atlanta, GA
BS Biochemistry
Magna Cum Laude

Honors and Awards

2013 **AOA**

2010 **Association of Pathology Chairs' Honor Society**
- Demonstrated academic excellence in pathology by receiving a course grade above 92% (16 students selected)

2009 **Arthur Ashe Award for Sports Scholars – First Team**
- One of eight NCAA tennis players to receive this award

2006–2009 **Dean's List**

2006–2009 **Academic All-American – Tennis**

2007 *ESPN The Magazine* **Academic All-District Second Team**

Extracurricular Activities

2012–present **Surgery Interest Group**
- Vice President

2010–present **BU Medical School Admissions**
- Committee member

2006–2010 **Emory University, Men's Varsity Tennis**
- Co-captain Division III NCAA men's national champions

Figure 8.3 CV Sample 3.

Work and Research Experience

2012–present   Lahey Clinic Department of Surgery
Laboratory Assistant, Dr. Peter Smith
- Evaluated the feasibility of implanting a novel percutaneously deployed LVAD in patients with cardiogenic shock

Professional Memberships

2012–present   American Medical Association

2012–present   American College of Physicians

Publications

Abstracts and Poster Presentations

Sfakianos A, **Jones S**, Smith P. *Implantation of a novel percutaneously deployed LVAD in a patient with medical refractory cardiogenic shock.* Annual Cardiothoracic Symposium. San Diego, CA. 2014.

Interests

Basketball, football, traveling, tennis, horology.

Chapter 8

Figure 8.3 (*continued*)

in Alpha Omega Alpha and All-American tennis status. Therefore, it was correct for this candidate to list the Honors and Awards and Extracurricular Activities sections immediately after the Education section. While the candidate does have some research experience and an abstract, listing this section on the second page was the wise thing to do.

Specific Comments

Comment 1

This CV does a nice job of highlighting the significance of the candidate's accomplishments. For example, Sam Jones received the Arthur Ashe Award. The significance of this may be lost upon the reviewer if he had not succinctly summarized it:

Arthur Ashe Award for Sports Scholars – First Team
One of eight NCAA tennis players to receive this award

As one of only eight tennis players in the nation to receive it, this award takes on more significance.

Comment 2

This CV used multiple abbreviations. The use of NCAA to describe the National Collegiate Athletic Association is acceptable, as most people may not even recognize the latter. One would hope that everyone in the medical field would recognize the abbreviation "AOA," yet it would have been better to write Alpha Omega Alpha to ensure that he received full credit for induction into this prestigious society. Technical abbreviations such as "LVAD" (left ventricular assist device) should also be defined.

Comment 3

The candidate lists horology as an interest. Remember that whatever you list on your CV can be discussed during an interview. The candidate better be able to discuss the watch that the interviewer is wearing, as he is sure to be asked many questions about horology.

References

1. Jackson, A. L. and Geckeis, K. C. (2003) *How to Prepare your Curriculum Vitae.* New York, NY: McGraw-Hill.
2. Katta, R. and Samir, D. (2009) *The Successful Match: 200 Rules to Succeed in the Residency Match.* Houston, TX: MD2B.
3. Kennedy, J. L. (2011) *Resumes for Dummies,* 6th edn. Hoboken, NJ: John Wiley & Sons, Inc.
4. Le, T., Bhushan, V., and Shenvi, C. (2010) *First Aid for the Match,* 5th edn. New York, NY: McGraw-Hill Medical.
5. Smith, R. P. (2000) *From Medical School to Residency: How to Compete Successfully in the Residency Match Program.* New York, NY: Springer.
6. Whitcomb, S. B. (2010) *Resume Magic,* 4th edn. Indianapolis, IN: JIST Publishing.
7. Eisenberg, R. L., Cunningham, M., Kung, J. W., and Slanetz, P. J. (2013) Misrepresentation of publications by radiology applicants: is it really a problem? *Journal of the American College of Radiology* **10** (3): 195–197.

9: The Personal Statement

The personal statement is one of the most daunting components of the application. It is one of the few portions of the application that is completely under your control and your one chance to "humanize" your application. Students recognize that a well-written personal statement will engage readers by allowing them insight into their personality and view of the world. Consequently, applicants often fret about presenting themselves in the best light. The role of the personal statement cannot be underestimated. The 2012 National Resident Matching Program (NRMP®) *Program Director Survey* [1] revealed that the personal statement was the third most commonly used factor in selecting whom to interview, trailing only the United States Medical Licensing Examination® (USMLE®) Step 1 score and letters of recommendation.

There is no "cookie-cutter" personal statement. However, a well-written personal statement should convey the following information:

- **Who you are.**
- **Your motivation for going into your chosen specialty.**
- **Desirable attributes which make you an asset to the program**. These can be generally sought-after traits such as enthusiasm, a solid work ethic, a conscientious nature, and a team spirit.
- **What you are looking for in a residency program**. Since you can upload program-specific personal statements to the Electronic Residency Application Service (ERAS®), you can emphasize characteristics that may be of unique interest at that program — such as a penchant for quality improvement at a program where the Chairman is a frequent speaker on that topic.
- **Your future goals.**

Applicants approach the task of writing an effective personal statement in a variety of ways, but the most common method is to weave a past event or outstanding skill into your narrative. Many students have had unique moments that have shaped their decision to enter their chosen field, such as the illness of a family member, taking care of a specific patient, or participating in a ground-breaking medical procedure. Others may have particular motivations for going into a specialty, such as the All-American athlete who is interested in Orthopedics. Use your statement to allow the reader to have a better understanding of your personal journey in medicine. Obviously, you have to be honest. Do not fabricate an epiphany or emotional experience just to pull at the heartstrings of the selection committee members. Any experience, no matter how small it may seem, that led you to your specialty of choice is an important story. Told in the right context, it can serve as the theme for your statement.

Insider Tip: Do not fabricate stories so that your personal statement reads better.

The personal statement also provides an opportunity to highlight some of your strongest achievements. This does not mean simply rehashing your curriculum vitae (CV). Instead, choose a few of your most impressive moments or extracurricular activities and highlight them prominently. Examples might include your role in establishing a student-run health clinic, or perhaps your experiences as a concert violinist or performing clinically significant research. Use this opportunity to show how your involvement in these activities has given you the necessary personal qualities to succeed in your chosen field. For general reading, see the References section [2–8].

The following pages give multiple **Insider Tips** about the personal statement, but the single most important advice is to start early, for it certainly will be one of the most time-consuming portions of your application. A good start date is late spring/early summer, so that you have sufficient time for showing it to others for input and to give you plenty of time to make revisions. Write a draft, which will likely be the first of many, and then let it simmer for a week or two. Chances are that your original version will go through drastic changes over the course of multiple drafts. Enlist the help of a trusted friend or family member to critique what you have written. It is a double-edged sword asking more than one or two close friends for help, for this may result in your being inundated with so many suggestions that your personal statement can quickly lose its "personal touch." When you are comfortable that you are near a final version, ask the opinion of your advisor, whose experience in this area can add valuable insight. Depending on how well you know the authors of your letters of recommendation, you can also give them a somewhat polished draft, along with your CV and ERAS form. They can give you valuable feedback, and what you have written may be a helpful guide for composing their own letters. Do not be frustrated if you have to start from scratch multiple times, for you certainly will not be the first or last applicant to do this.

Insider Tip: The most important advice for writing a personal statement is to start early. A well-written personal statement goes through many iterations before the final product, and you want to leave sufficient time to clear your head between each version.

Addressing Flaws/Gaps in the Application

Before moving on to additional insider tips, a special word about addressing "red flags" in your application. If you have a significant flaw or gap in your application, such as a very low USMLE Step 1 score, a portion of the personal statement can be used to address this issue. For example, perhaps an illness or recent passage of a loved one affected your performance. On rare occasions, a subpar USMLE Step 1 score did not meet our threshold, but an explanation in the personal statement made us reconsider the candidate's other merits more closely. A large gap in your work/education timeline is also important to address, because failure to do so may lead program directors to the conclusion that you have suffered from a psychiatric illness. Other potential "red flags," such as being a non-traditional student, can be skillfully discussed and turned from concerns into attributes. For example, if you are an older student, your maturity could be seen as a valuable attribute if spun correctly. If you have taken time off, stress how the experience and development of a skill set outside of medicine represent important attributes.

If you do plan on addressing a difficult issue on your application, it is important to spend sufficient time thinking about how best to go about doing this. Make sure that you accept responsibility for the problem and discuss how it helped you to develop as a physician and a person. Do not make excuses for your failures, for no one likes to work with someone who takes this approach. For example, the following are two statements from candidates who fared poorly on their General Surgery rotation:

Statement I

Finally, I would like to address my grade of Pass on General Surgery. I suffered a loss in my immediate family one week prior to the Shelf examination. The stress of the situation and travel before my examination contributed to my low score. I hope that the committee will consider my scores on the remainder of my clinical rotations as a demonstration of my true academic potential.

Statement II

Finally, I would like to address my grade of Pass on General Surgery, as I suffered a loss in my immediate family one week prior to the Shelf examination. This experience taught me the importance of managing my personal and work life and, in retrospect, I should have considered postponing my test. I hope that the committee will consider my scores on the remainder of my clinical rotations as a demonstration of my true academic potential.

Notice that both candidates have very similar statements. Candidate I blames his low score on stress and travel, which is likely completely accurate. However, stating that stress and travel attributed to his poor performance is probably not a good idea, given that stress is inherently associated with all of the medical specialties. Candidate II mentions the loss of a family member and gives a somewhat cryptic response about managing personal and work life, but makes no further excuse for his low score. Both then proceed to point out their successes on the remainder of their clinical rotations. Candidate II presents a better approach of addressing a suboptimal result by accepting responsibility and explaining how the experience helped them grow as a physician.

More Insider Tips for the Personal Statement

- **The opening paragraph is by far the most important one and must "hook" the reader.** After all, program directors read hundreds or even thousands of personal statements each year. To really stand out, your statement has to grab their attention right from the beginning. Here is an example of a good opening:

    "All of you students should look at this head CT and appreciate that last night one of our second-year radiology residents likely saved this patient's life." The four students on Neuroradiology at that time all intently looked at the image, hoping to identify the pathology.

    After you have hooked the reader, each individual paragraph in the remainder of your statement should be centered about a specific topic, such as why you believe the specialty is appropriate for you and what your future plans are in the field. This will allow program directors to understand your motivations for applying to a residency in their specialty. Your last paragraph should end strongly and tie everything together.

- **Your personal statement should fit on one page, so it is important to be concise and make every sentence count.** To this end, it is important to write in an active rather than passive voice. For those of you who have never read or forgotten to read Strunk and White's *The Elements of Style* [6], here are a few examples of active versus passive sentences:

Chapter 9

Active
1. *The medical student performed the procedure flawlessly.*
2. *The patient held the student's hand tightly during the procedure.*

Passive
1. *The procedure was performed flawlessly by the medical student.*
2. *The student's hand was held tightly by the patient during the procedure.*

Notice that in an active sentence, the subject acts upon the verb. In a passive sentence, the subject is acted upon by the verb. Active sentences are more concise.

- **Do not "stick your neck out" and submit an unorthodox essay.** Personal statements are rarely game changers. Do not submit an unorthodox personal statement, such as a poem or song. Stick to the playbook on the personal statement.

- **Do not overstate your credentials.** Do not exaggerate the importance of your projects or your role working on them. Interviewers know that as a medical student you were not the driving force behind the creation of an artificial heart or a breakthrough in stem cell technology. Thanks to the internet, it is very easy to verify any awards, accolades, or publications that you list.

- **Do not use your medical school admissions essay.** Personal statements too often are rooted in the early and undergraduate years. Residency directors are interested in your growth during medical school and how that has shaped your decision to enter the field. Do not simply rehash your medical school admissions essay.

- **Avoid discussion of politics and religion.** Avoid controversial topics in your statement, particularly "third rail" topics such as politics and religion. With half the country voting one way and the other half the opposite way, you are almost certain to offend someone. In general, incendiary or controversial topics should not be broached.

- **Avoid clichés.** Do not use clichés in your writing. It demonstrates laziness and lack of creativity. The following are examples:
  1. *My experience taking care of Mr. Smith taught me that **time heals all wounds**.*
  2. *After experiencing firsthand the recovery of 5-year-old Jon, I was reminded that **laughter is the best medicine**.*

- **Edit your personal statement carefully!** Grammatical errors on a personal statement can be a kiss of death to your application, especially if you are a foreign medical graduate. Run spell-check multiple times, but remember that a correct spelling of an incorrect word will not be detected. Always make sure to have several people read through it.

- **Do not go over one page!** The review committee reads hundreds of applications, and they are turned off by applicants who write too much. As a result, use direct and concrete sentences, and do not ramble. Make sure that everything flows smoothly together and is not choppy; it may help to read it aloud to identify the transitions. Start and end strong – you want to immediately grab the attention of your readers and leave them with a tight, unifying finish.

- **Review sample personal statements.** The internet is littered with these and many medical schools will also provide samples of well-written personal statements.

Samples 1 and 2 (Figures 9.1 and 9.2, respectively) present a few examples of personal statements.

My parents named me after the tiny village in which I grew up: Yi-ling. Ling means serenity, and it aptly described my hometown, nestled deep in the lush forests of southern China. I spent much of my childhood in an austere environment without electricity or running water, where healthcare was a luxury reserved only for emergencies. Today, only a few nostalgic neurons still retain memories of those wonder years. My most prominent, feature me slumped on my mother's back, feverish and weak as she trekked to the hospital 5 miles away on foot. I was a sickly child, and this was a regular occurrence. I grew to hate those sterile white walls and the often anguished look on my mother's face. I felt helpless against my own body as my nascent mind could not grasp why illnesses occurred. My immigration to the US at 11 marked a change in this dynamic; almost fittingly, I became enthralled by biology and the cellular processes that governed our existence. My research and volunteer experiences in college proved that not all suffering was insurmountable and, as I was no longer a child, I firmly chose to pursue medicine.

This pursuit has been an inspirational and humbling journey. During my first two years, I was always fascinated by imaging modalities that lent tantalizing glimpses into internal anatomical structures. After a year on the wards, what began as an interest in radiology grew into a passion as I saw how heavily clinicians relied on imaging to make diagnoses. The intellectual challenges inherent in the field were particularly alluring, as they required a breadth of knowledge that spanned all specialties. Just as my research demanded critical analysis, radiology requires me to systematically evaluate objective imaging data in the context of my two favorite subjects, anatomy and pathology. Knowing the clinical manifestations of the disease, condensing the underlying pathophysiology, and watching the shadows it casts onto visualizable images call for a particular kind of observational talent. The meticulous search for seemingly unrelated abnormalities and the ability to correlate them to the patient's history to make a diagnosis is an immensely gratifying process - detective work akin to that of Sherlock Holmes, my first hero in Western literature. The inductive reasoning so prominently featured in radiology intrigues me and I aspire to become a master sleuth in medicine. Finally, radiologists are pivotal to the team-based approach to medicine. In total, my strength and interests all align - I value the chance to work closely with my clinician colleagues and assemble the clues for them from strong objective data for their diagnosis and management of patients.

Residency will be crucial for my growth as a physician, and a program that offers comprehensive training through a variety of pathology in an encouraging environment will promote the most growth. Since I learn best through experience, a large volume of disparate imaging findings will build the strongest foundation for my future career and prepare my way for fellowship after residency. In addition, I hope to find inspiring mentors and teachers who will guide me in my training and provide advice regarding matters both in and out of the field. Paired with a strong resident camaraderie and culture, this support will allow me to reach new heights. Finally, I seek a program that embraces technological advancements and provides a supportive environment for resident research. As technology continues to evolve and revolutionize medicine, I want to be on the cutting edge for future diagnostic and therapeutic breakthroughs.

In retrospect, I have grown so much from that naïve and helpless child living in rural China. From a life without running water to a career defined by technology, these opportunities in America have transformed my life. Finishing residency will give me the chance to finally put my knowledge and skills to work and give back to a world that has been so kind to me. As I stand a step closer to my goal, I look forward to joining a program that will hone my skills to Holmesian levels, and allow me to work with a team of physicians to provide the highest level of care for our patients.

Figure 9.1 Personal statement: Sample 1.

Both literally and figuratively, running has taken me far. It took me three thousand miles away from my home in Boston to California for my undergraduate education and from there, all over the country and beyond for competitions. Because of running, I have met the President of the United States in his own home and built some of my most valued relationships over a shared interest in the sport. All through medical school, however, I have fought my identity as a runner, assuming instead, that which I thought should belong to a medical student and future doctor. My third year felt like a roller coast, as I attempted to fully immerse myself in each field. I learned to appreciate the unexpected turns in the life of an obstetrician, embrace the adrenaline rushes experienced as a surgeon, and endure, at times, the long flat stretches of time on an internal medicine day. As fourth year began, I realized that that an identity as a runner is not mutually exclusive with that of a physician. What makes me feel grounded, in fact, is what has made me a good athlete and, I believe, will make for a successful career in orthopedic surgery.

I have long known orthopedic surgery was the perfect fit for me. As an athlete, I have been exposed first hand to numerous sports related injuries and have admired orthopedic surgeons for their ability to precisely diagnosis ailments through physical exam and then correct them through surgical intervention. An orthopedic surgeon must be able to work in a multidisciplinary environment interacting with internists, radiologists, and anesthesiologists, as well as spend hours independently in the operating room.

My career as a runner has instilled in me the personal attributes which I believe will help me in the field of orthopedic surgery. Through countless hours of training, I have learned to work well independently and remain self motivated. At the same, time, my running career has allowed me to participate in a team sport with wonderful teammates. My year as co-captain of an NCAA championship track team taught me the importance of teamwork and mentoring my younger teammates who were world-class athletes, but who were not used to the rigors of collegiate athletics. Finally, my career as a marathoner, taught me the importance of perseverance. While my times have ranged from a top ten finish in the Chicago Marathon, to well out of the top one hundred finishers, I have always completed my race.

While excitement and passion for orthopedic surgery is not something unique to me among an impressive pool of applicants, the program that inherits me, will be gaining a resident dedicated to her patients, loyal to her colleagues, and insistent on only the best of herself and of those who surround her. My ideal program is one that establishes high expectations and challenges its residents, but teaches with understanding and patience. I can see myself one day focusing my attention on female athletes, particularly those with hip dysfunction.

My journey through medical school has represented a shift from competitive athlete to medical student and recreational jogger. While I have been exposed to a variety of specialties, I have ultimately chosen to stick to the ground I am most familiar with and pursue a career in orthopedic surgery, a field I believe suits my personality and interests best.

Figure 9.2 Personal statement: Sample 2.

Comments on Sample 1

General comments.

This statement is interesting to read because the applicant has an unusual path and shares her personal journey into medicine and eventually diagnostic radiology. The applicant uses her life story as a unifying theme. There are no grammatical or spelling errors, which is important since the applicant is not originally from the United States.

Specific Comments

Comment 1

This personal statement is well organized and has a unifying theme. The opening paragraph immediately grabs the reader's attention and each following paragraph is centered around its own theme. Paragraph 1 allows the reader insight into the factors that shaped the applicant's life. Paragraph 2 explains why the applicant is interested in radiology. Paragraph 3 explains what she is looking for in a residency program. Paragraph 4 ties the essay together.

Comment 2

This essay is one page. It is important to limit your essay to one page and four or five paragraphs. The second paragraph is long and thus a bit intimidating in appearance. Try to keep your individual paragraphs at a manageable length.

Comment 3

One aspect that this essay lacks is concrete evidence of specific achievements that the applicant has accomplished. She mentions research, but does not give any details about research accomplishments or projects.

Comments on Sample 2

General comments

This is a well written personal statement. We are presented with a clear reason why the candidate is interested in orthopedic surgery and she is able to integrate running as a unifying theme throughout the narrative.

Specific Comments

Comment 1

This personal statement is well organized and has a unifying theme. The paragraphs are a bit shorter than the first sample, making it easier to read.

Comment 2

This personal statement differs from Sample 1 in that the writer is able to integrate her considerable achievements into the essay. Note that the personal statement should not simply rehash your CV. However, if you have significant achievements that you would like to highlight, the personal statement offers another opportunity to do so. This applicant was able to integrate their accomplishments with the essence of the narrative.

Comment 3

It is important to mention the specialty to which you are applying within the first two paragraphs. The first sample personal statement mentions medicine in the opening paragraph, but only in the second paragraph does the reader realize that the writer is applying to Radiology. In the second sample, it is clear after reading the first paragraph that the applicant is applying to Orthopedic Surgery.

Chapter 9

References

1. NRMP (2012) *National Resident Matching Program, Data Release and Research Committee: Results of the 2012 NRMP Program Director Survey.* Washington, DC: National Resident Matching Program.

2. Katta, R. and Samir, D. (2009) *The Successful Match: 200 Rules to Succeed in the Residency Match.* Houston, TX: MD2B.

3. Kennedy, J. L. (2011) *Resumes for Dummies*, 6th edn. Hoboken, NJ: John Wiley & Sons, Inc.

4. Le, T., Bhushan, V., and Shenvi, C. (2010) *First Aid for the Match*, 5th edn. New York, NY: McGraw-Hill Medical.

5. Smith, R. P. (2000) *From Medical School to Residency: How to Compete Successfully in the Residency Match Program.* New York, NY: Springer.

6. Strunk, W., Jr. and White, E. B. (2009) *The Elements of Style*, 5th edn. Boston, MA: Allyn & Bacon.

7. American Medical Student Association – Essentials of getting into a surgical residency; available from: http://www.amsa.org/AMSA/Libraries/Committee_Docs/Essentials_of_a_Getting_into_a_Surgical_Residency.sflb.ashx [accessed June 2014].

8. American Medical Association – Writing your personal statement; available from: http://www.ama-assn.org/ama/pub/about-ama/our-people/member-groups-sections/minority-affairs-section/transitioning-residency/writing-your-personal-statement.page [accessed June 2014].

10: The Interview

You have finally got it – the coveted interview invitation. The countless hours spent writing your personal statement and filling out your Electronic Residency Application Service (ERAS®) application have paid off. But do not sit back and rest on your laurels. No matter how strong a candidate you are on paper, for many programs, the interview is the single most important factor in the selection process. The 2012 National Resident Matching Program (NRMP®) *Program Director Survey* [1] revealed that, besides being flagged for a match violation, the interview and interaction with the faculty was the most important factor in deciding how to rank a candidate. For most programs, a bad interview is a deal-breaker.

As a candidate, you have two major goals entering the interview. First, you must convince your interviewers that they can work with you for the next few years and that you will fit into the culture of the program. Remember that you have been issued an invitation because the program feels that you have the necessary academic credentials to succeed. However, this is true for all of the candidates who were invited to interview. During your interview, you must demonstrate that you have the necessary social skills to be a successful member of the medical team. Your second goal during the interview is to find out as much information as you can about the program, so you can decide whether it would be a good fit for you. Residency training is not easy, which makes it all the more important for you to like the program where you are training.

In this chapter, we will guide you through the interview process by breaking it down into a few basic steps: interview preparation, a typical interview day, and interview pitfalls. With a little preparation and a few tips, you will ace the interview. For general reading, see the References section [2–5].

Preparing for the Interview

In many ways, preparing for the interview is almost as important as the interview itself. Provisional steps include scheduling an interview, choosing an appropriate outfit, planning what to bring, performing due diligence researching the program, and conducting mock interviews.

Scheduling Your Interview

The interview season typically runs from October through January. Programs offer interviews either on a rolling basis or as bulk invitations. You can expect most invitations to be through email or ERAS. In some specialties, such as Ophthalmology, interview invitations can sometimes be issued by telephone. It is important to respond promptly. At our program, interview dates are booked within *1 week* of sending out invitations. Thus, you must respond immediately and reserve a date, even if it is not ideal for you. Occasionally, it is possible to choose another date outside those offered, especially late in the interview season when applicants begin cancelling interviews. However, do not stall in making this determination. Email the program coordinator promptly with your request. Keep in close touch with the program coordinator, but avoid being a pest.

> **Insider Tip:** After getting an invitation for an interview, do not delay scheduling it.

There is a debate about whether it is better to schedule interviews with your most coveted programs early or late. Some believe that doing well on an early interview sets the bar high for subsequent applicants and can help you stand out. These proponents for early interviews believe that candidates tend to burn out during later ones. Others are convinced that early candidates are often forgotten, with later applicants more likely to stand out in the interviewers' minds. Later applicants tend to be more confident and polished than those who interview earlier. Having interviewed for several years, we believe that both lines of reasoning are true. You must have a truly great interview if your intention is to set a high bar early. Most candidates are solid, but not great interviewees. If this is your situation, scheduling your most coveted programs for the middle to latter portion of the interview season may be the wisest move. In any case, you should definitely have a few interviews under your belt before visiting your top choices. If you do have an early interview at a favored program, send them an email near the end of their interview cycle to remind them of your interest, so that your application is fresh in their mind.

When scheduling interviews, remember to pace yourself. Try to avoid scheduling too many in one week, especially if they are on different coasts. A typical interview is 2 days, with a dinner the night before the formal interview day. Although it is ideal if you can group your interviews by city, such as traveling to Boston one week and Los Angeles the next, this is often not realistic given the differences between interview dates and invitations. If you are going to be in the area and wish to either switch a date or have not yet heard back from the program, make contact with them. If it is simply a matter of changing dates, work with the program coordinator. However, if a desired program has not yet invited you for an interview, politely mention your travel plans and ask whether they have already sent out the bulk of their invitations. If they have done so, back off – you do not want to be a pest while they consider filling cancellation spots. Consider sending additional application materials about recent accomplishments or clerkship grades. Another approach is to request that an advisor or other faculty member make a phone call on your behalf. If you are lucky enough to land an interview but absolutely cannot make the date and the coordinator has no other open slots to offer, some candidates resort to arranging a switch with another candidate. Interview blog sites are often used. For instance, some radiology applicants use www.auntminnie.com to arrange internal date switches and then notify the program. We do *not* recommend doing this for any program that you covet, as the reaction of a program to this approach is unpredictable.

While on the topic of travel, there is an enormous financial burden placed upon applicants, especially those who must also interview for Preliminary and Transitional Year spots in addition to residency programs. The cost of travel to interviews can be prohibitive, as financial aid packages for your fourth year do not reflect this additional expense. Therefore, some students apply for GradPLUS or private loans to ease application travel expenses. Other candidates, particularly those applying regionally, find the cost more manageable by employing thrifty measures such as using discount travel sites (www.kayak.com, www .priceline.com, or www.orbitz.com) or frequent flyer miles, or by building up travel points with a credit card reward program. Lesser-known housing options include school-specific programs, through which an alumnus hosts an applicant, or discounted housing offered by a residency program.

Choosing an Appropriate Outfit

Your interview is definitely no time for a fashion experiment. If you have an alternative or edgy look, hide it. Men should wear a navy or gray, solid or pinstripe suit and a tie. A pressed, long-sleeved, white or blue shirt is appropriate. Avoid wearing bowties, earrings, or jewelry. Short, clean-cut hair is preferred; goatees are less desirable. There is a Chinese proverb that "the tallest tree is the first to be chopped down." Similarly, when in doubt, choose the more conservative option and blend in with the crowd.

Women have wider latitude, but business attire is appropriate. A skirt suit is often the clothing of choice, but a blouse and pants suit or a conservative dress is fine as well. Skirts should be knee length and be prepared for snagged stockings by having an extra pair in your purse. Jewelry should be understated. Body piercings (other than in the ears) should be removed. Makeup should be applied tastefully. Perfume should be omitted or used very sparingly. If you wear nail polish, apply standard colors. For example, one candidate to our program wore black nail polish, which was the subject of comments from multiple interviewers.

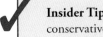

Insider Tip: Never let your clothes or accessories be the focus of an interview. Dress conservatively!

Planning What to Bring

If you are flying to an interview, try to fit everything into a carry-on bag (Box 10.1) to eliminate the risk of lost luggage. Carry or wear your suit on the airplane. You do not want to be dressed in jeans during your interviews. On interview day, many candidates carry a leather portfolio binder with them. We have rarely seen anyone open one, but it seems to give candidates a sense of comfort. While most interviewers have seen your application, it is possible that someone may be filling in at the last moment. Therefore, we recommend carrying with you a copy of your curriculum vitae (CV) and any important scientific papers that you have written.

Box 10.1 Travel Checklist.

Plane tickets	Deodorant
Suit and tie	Comb
Shirts (2)	Floss
Shoes	Cell phone and charger
Undergarments	Printout of interview day schedule
Money	Printout of directions to medical center
Toothbrush and toiletries	Umbrella/overcoat

Perform Due Diligence

Before you interview, research the program thoroughly. Revisit the notes you made about the program when making your application list, and look again at the department's website to refresh your memory. The website often conveys the tone and mission of the program, which can help you tailor your presentation appropriately. Use this information to formulate a few program-specific questions, which will send the message that you are truly interested in training there.

Make sure that you visit the specialty-specific websites. Medical student chat forums often have very useful information about specific programs. It is also helpful to speak to any former residents or faculty members you may know who have trained there. They can give you the inside scoop. If those residents or faculty members are well regarded, feel free to "name drop" during an interview.

Just as knowing about a program is valuable, knowing something about your interviewers is equally important. While it is difficult to predict exactly which staff will conduct interviews, it is a safe bet that the Program Director and Associate Program Directors will be meeting with you. Other potential interviewers include the Chairman, Director of Medical Student Education and the chief residents. While having in-depth knowledge about the personal lives of interviewers is not necessary (do not be a stalker), some basic knowledge about their training and research focus is helpful, especially if you have common interests that can be emphasized. At the very least, be able to recognize the names of the Program Director and Associate Program Directors. Nothing starts an interview off on the wrong foot more than a candidate asking a Program Director what their role in the department is!

Insider Tip: Perform due diligence by knowing some details about your interviewers ahead of time.

Do not forget that every aspect of your record is fair game during an interview. So you must know your application thoroughly. Go through every portion of your CV and be able to speak intelligently and authoritatively about all aspects of it. Now is the time to refresh yourself on the protein kinase C pathway that you wrote about 8 years ago and the abstract that you presented as a college student. Interviewers often focus on the most obscure elements of your CV and expect you to speak knowledgeably about them. For example, one candidate listed gift wrapping as an interest. Her interviewer brought in wrapping paper and watched as she wrapped a Christmas present for him!

> **Insider Tip:** Perform due diligence on yourself!

You should also use this time to re-evaluate your record for holes that may be probed by interviewers. These include unexplained absences, poor grades, and non-traditional pathways to medicine. While it is never desirable to be in a position to explain such things, remember that the program must regard you highly since you have already been selected for an interview. It is best to accept responsibility for a poor result and demonstrate how it has helped you grow as a person and physician. For example, if questioned about a "Pass" grade in Medicine, one could respond:

> I was initially very surprised by my grade in Medicine, but I ultimately believe that it helped me become a better physician. I met with my attending physician and senior resident and they gave me constructive criticism. I was able to apply that to my remaining rotations, in all of which I received a grade of Honors or High Pass. Most importantly, I was able to improve my clinical skills through their advice.

Similarly, if you took a circuitous route to medicine, your life experience could be a positive asset:

> My four years as a consultant at McKinsey provided me with the opportunity to travel the country and interact with a wide range of personalities. I believe that the experiences that I have gained have been valuable during medical school and will continue to help me throughout my medical career.

Finally, make sure that you have reviewed your digital footprint. By this we mean search for current or old Facebook, Instagram, and other accounts and lock or preferably delete them. In one *JAMA* article [2], 60% of US medical schools reported incidents of students posting unprofessional content online [6]. Do not assume that your Facebook account is off limits for Program Directors to view.

Conduct a Mock Interview

Similar to other skills in life, becoming a good interviewee takes practice. Do not assume that your pleasant personality will automatically translate into being a good interviewee. It is important to practice with anyone who will listen, such as trusted classmates, friends, and family. When you are feeling confident, schedule a mock interview with an advisor or through the Office of Student Affairs at your medical school [7].

Approach a mock interview as you would an official one, dressing in your formal interview outfit. Before your interview, your number one priority is to make sure that you have a plan about how to cohesively present why you will be a valuable member of the medical team and will fit in well. By the end of the session, your interviewer should understand what makes you a good candidate, what makes you unique, and how these attributes will help you integrate into their program.

The best interviewees are engaging. They tend to be relaxed and excellent conversationalists, who use a combination of sense of humor, non-verbal gestures, excellent listening skills, and thoughtful answers to navigate their way through the interview. While not all candidates, or interviewers for that matter, have the personality and sense of humor to achieve this level of interview proficiency, there are certain aspects of your social interaction and answer content that can be corrected during your practice interviews.

Make sure to work on your greeting. The decision about a candidate is often made during the first few minutes of an interview and your introduction can play a large role. Greet your interviewers with a smile and a firm handshake, looking them in the eye when you introduce yourself. Address all interviewers by their formal titles (e.g., Dr. Smith). If your hands get sweaty, keep them on your lap or in your pockets along with a pair of tissues, so that you can wipe them prior to shaking hands. Take your cue of where and when to sit from your interviewer.

Non-verbal gestures, such as posture, are extremely important. Sit up straight and look the interviewer in the eye. Though it may seem strange to mention, occasionally break eye contact. An applicant in our most recent interview cycle made his interviewers uncomfortable by leaning into all questions and seemingly never blinking. Keep your hands folded on your lap for the majority of the interview, using hand gestures when necessary. Avoid resting on the interviewer's desk or the back of the chair, as this can be misconstrued as disrespect rather than a relaxed manner. It is important to appear attentive and engaged, even if you could not care less about what the interviewer is saying.

Rehearse your answers to commonly asked interview questions prior to your interview (Box 10.2). The ideal answer is neither too long nor short, but to the point. Make sure that you sound sincere and not too polished. It is not good if the interviewers think of you as a used car salesman.

You should also have a list of questions to ask your interviewer (Box 10.3). Generally, it is recommended that you ask "safe questions" that keep the mood of the interview upbeat. For example, if there is a new Chairwoman in the department, asking about faculty turnover may not be the best idea. Similarly, do not ask questions that can be easily answered by simply clicking on the program's website. For example, a Program Director who has established a well-known international public health rotation may not appreciate the candidate asking whether there are opportunities to take a rotation abroad. Questions regarding salary, benefits, vacation,

Box 10.2 Commonly Asked Interview Questions.

Why did you choose your specialty?
Why are you interested in this program?
Tell me about yourself
What is your greatest strength/weakness?
What can you contribute to our program?
Where do you see yourself in 10 years?
What is the biggest challenge facing our specialty/medicine?
What do you do in your spare time?
What was the most interesting case you were involved with?
Tell me about this item on your CV
If you were not doing this specialty, what specialty/other occupation would you choose?
How do you handle difficult situations?
Describe an embarrassing situation and how you handled it

Box 10.3 Questions to Ask the Interviewer.

What is the greatest strength/weakness of the program?
What is one thing that you would change about your program?
How is your department's relationship with other services?
Do residents go on to fellowships?
Do all faculty participate in teaching?
What do you look for in a candidate?
Are there research opportunities?
Do you foresee any changes within the department?

Box 10.4 Questions *Not* to Ask the Interviewer.

What is the salary?
What are the benefits?
What is the vacation time?
Is there maternity leave?

and maternity leave are best left to investigating on the website or by contacting the Graduate Medical Education office at the hospital (Box 10.4).

Just as you practiced your greeting, make sure that you spend an equal amount of time rehearsing your closing. Similar to your greeting, stand up straight, look your interviewer in the eye, and shake hands firmly. Your objective is both to thank them and to convey your continued interest in the program. A typical closing statement may be:

> Thank you so much for taking the time to interview me. I just wanted to emphasize again how impressed I am with your program and how honored I would be to have the opportunity to train here.

Typical Interview Day

The interview is an opportunity for the program to attach a face to your application, as well as for you to learn more about the program. In some cases, programs view all applicants as equal entering the interview. In others, programs have pre-ranked candidates and have preferences that the interview is designed to confirm or reject. Whatever your status going in, you do not want your interview to be the factor that drops you to the bottom of their rank list. Unfortunately, that may well happen. We have had highly regarded candidates from top medical schools go from being highly competitive to the "Do Not Rank" list, based solely on a poor interview. Conversely, candidates from lesser-ranked schools have moved to the top of our list on the basis of their interviews.

The interview day is long and often comprised of many facets, including interviews with multiple members of the selection committee, a tour of the department, and a meal, with some interviews beginning the night before with a social event. These pre-interview socials are usually attended by current residents, while at some programs faculty may be present as well. No matter how casual the setting, do not forget that these events constitute part of the interview process. Resident dinners are a great chance for the program to evaluate you in a social situation and gauge your interaction with current residents. Avoid inappropriate topics, jokes, or foul language. Do not become inebriated. If you do not normally drink, do not order anything alcoholic to calm nerves or try to fit in. It may go straight to your head. If you do normally drink alcohol and the resident attendees are drinking, consider buying one drink and nursing it all night. Similarly, pay attention to what your fellow candidates are doing in terms of ordering food. Most programs pay for the dinner out of educational funds. While it is not necessary to just have a soup, do not order a three-course meal or the most expensive item on the menu, especially if everyone else is eating a sandwich. During the subsequent formal interview day, programs often ask the residents who attended the dinner about any odd or inappropriate conduct. Bad behavior can cause a candidate to be dead on arrival.

> **Insider Tip:** Pre-interview socials are absolutely part of the interview process, so try to attend and be on your best behavior.

The formal interview schedule typically runs for a full or half day. If a program tells you that the day ends around 5 p.m., the earliest you should plan on booking your outbound flight is 7 p.m., since you do not want to give the impression that you are not interested by hurrying off to the airport. During the visit, applicants are usually exposed to a didactic conference, tour of the department, lunch with the residents and/or faculty, and individual interviews. Interviewers typically include the Program Directors, faculty involved in the selection process, and one or two residents, most often the chief residents. However, the structure of the dedicated interviews varies, with some programs conducting panel interviews or asking you to perform specific tasks. For example, in the surgical specialties, candidates are occasionally asked to suture or carve a bar of soap as a means of testing hand–eye coordination. In general, most interviews are one-on-one and last 15–30 minutes each.

At the end of the day, interviewers meet to compare notes and rank candidates. They may actively solicit opinions from everyone you have met, from the program coordinators to your tour guides and other residents. Each program may focus on different attributes, but all are evaluating you during the interview and asking themselves whether they can envision working with you for the next few years. Showing disrespect to any of your future co-workers is a sure-fire way to convince them otherwise. At the wrap-up on our last interview day, an applicant was moved down the rank list because his tour guide informed us that he stayed at the back of the tour group yet talked so loudly and incessantly that other applicants had a hard time hearing the information. While not all opinions count equally, a bad interaction with a resident or even a program coordinator can derail an applicant's chances substantially.

> ✓ **Insider Tip:** The interview begins at your first contact with the program and ends with your last.

Interview Pitfalls: More Insider Tips

While it is true that most interviewers are not out to trick you, you should be aware of common interview pitfalls. Prior knowledge of these situations will help you avoid stumbling, as you will most likely encounter at least one of these potential pitfalls during your interview season.

- **When the interviewer asks you if you have any questions for him/her, make sure to ask one!** Usually, when the interviewer asks you whether you have any questions, it is a sign that the interview is nearing its end. When posed with this question, you *must* ask a question. A response such as "All of my questions were answered already" or "I do not have any more questions" is the *wrong* answer. Even if every question you had was answered already, you can always ask the same question to different interviewers. Not asking a question conveys a lack of interest to your interviewer.
- **Know how to approach "illegal questions."** Unfortunately, it is very likely that you will encounter an illegal question during one of your interviews. A survey of all US medical school graduates applying into Internal Medicine, General Surgery, Orthopedic Surgery, Obstetrics and Gynecology, and Emergency Medicine revealed that 65% of the respondents were asked at least one illegal question about gender, age, marital status, family, religion, ethnicity, or sexual orientation [8]. Questions related to marital status or children were most commonly asked and more often directed towards women. In an effort to combat illegal questions, the NRMP and the Council of Medical Specialty Societies Organization of Program Director Associations

have created a match code of conduct outlining proper conduct during the interview and match process. It specifically states that interviewers must refrain from asking questions regarding age, gender, religion, sexual orientation, and family status. Interviewers also cannot inquire about ranking preferences or the names of other institutions to which the candidate has applied.

There are three approaches to respond to an illegal question. The first is to either refuse to answer it or be confrontational. Although this choice is perfectly within your rights, it is not advised since it will probably result in your not matching at the program. For many illegal questions, providing a direct answer is a perfectly reasonable approach:

Interviewer: Are you married?

Answer: *No.*

For some questions, however, an honest answer may hurt your ranking:

Interviewer: Are you planning on having children during residency?

Answer: *Yes.*

If your interviewer is asking you such a question it is very possible that your answer may be considered during the ranking sessions. Thus, being completely honest in answering an illegal question may not always be the ideal approach.

The third option is to indirectly answer an interviewer's illegal question:

Interviewer: Are you planning on having children during residency?

Answer: *My husband and I are planning to eventually have children, and I think that family life helps one stay grounded. My main goal during my residency, however, is to learn the skills necessary to be a clinically excellent ophthalmologist and to contribute to the residency program.*

- **Stayed poised during the silent portions.** There may be a point where your interviewer remains silent for an extended period. Do not panic! Your interviewer may be employing a commonly used tactic to see how confident you are in your answer or simply just be thinking about what he/she will be having for lunch. Whatever the case, during this situation retain eye contact and continue smiling.

- **Do not stay too long or come too early.** It is hard to know how long is too long to stay on an interview day. Candidates often request to meet with additional faculty or tour facilities for which they have a particular interest. This is definitely a good way to show interest in a program, as well as an excellent opportunity to evaluate whether a certain program can fulfill your needs. But be wary of staying too long. An interview day is stressful enough for program coordinators. Accommodating additional requests just adds to their burden. Similarly, arrive at your interview 15 minutes early, but not before then. Your interviewers are busy clinicians who have tight schedules that do not account for unforeseen issues. In short, do not diverge too far from your interview schedule!

- **Understand that there are different interview styles.** Do not get too nervous if one of your interviewers is being overly aggressive or, alternatively, seems too casual. Similarly, do not become too confident if an interviewer is effusively praising you. Every interviewer has a different style, which may be intentionally preconceived. Some programs are known to have a "recruiter," whose task is to leave you with a very good feeling about the program. Some interviewers may be more confrontational, just to ensure that you can maintain composure under stress. If you are interviewing with someone who seems to be on one of these extremes, make sure you are on guard. Candidates often fall into the trap of revealing too much when an interviewer acts very informally, ending up shooting themselves in the foot.
- **Avoid eating foods that stain during lunch.** While this may sound silly, avoid foods that can stain your clothes, including ketchup, spaghetti, and mustard.

References

1. NRMP (2012) *Data Release and Research Committee: Results of the 2012 NRMP Program Director Survey.* Washington, DC: National Resident Matching Program.
2. Katta, R. and Samir, D. (2009) *The Successful Match: 200 Rules to Succeed in the Residency Match.* Houston, TX: MD2B.
3. Le, T., Bhushan, V., and Shenvi, C. (2010) *First Aid for the Match*, 5th edn. New York, NY: McGraw-Hill Medical.
4. Smith, R. P. (2000) *From Medical School to Residency: How to Compete Successfully in the Residency Match Program.* New York, NY: Springer.
5. Freedman, J. (2010) *The Residency Interview: How to Make the Best Possible Impression.* Los Angeles, CA: MedEdits Publishing.
6. Chretien, K. C., *et al.* (2009) Online posting of unprofessional content by medical students. *JAMA* **302** (12): 1309–1315.
7. American Medical Association – Mock-residency interview; available from: http://www.ama-assn.org/resources/doc/img/mock-residency-interview.pdf [accessed June 2014].
8. Hern, H. G., Jr., *et al.* (2013) How prevalent are potentially illegal questions during residency interviews? *Academic Medicine* **88** (8): 1116–1121.

11: After the Interview

Now that the interview is over, you can exhale and pat yourself on the back. You are over the application hump, but your job is not yet finished. You still have to develop your rank list for submission by late February. Our admission committee at Beth Israel Deaconess Medical Center, like many others, meets immediately after interviews to rank candidates. Thus, your preliminary rank position is set before you even step foot on the airplane taking you back home. But there is a lot of time between the interview and the *final* rank meeting …

How to Improve

After the interview, your first order of business is to review the day's events and consider ways to improve. For instance:

- **Were you late?** This is a pretty big no-no, but if you were late, hopefully you were profusely apologetic and avoided lame excuses. You are an adult and know how to be on time, but when punctuality is so important it is necessary to take extra measures. Consider battery-operated backup alarms and hotel wakeup calls. If you are in the area the night before, map out a route to your interview location, including parking garages. If it is a very large hospital, consider locating the exact room where you will meet. The morning of an interview, check traffic-sensitive GPS maps for the best route and give yourself plenty of travel time. If you get there early, hang out in the lobby until 15 minutes before your scheduled arrival time rather than hovering around the desk of a busy Program Coordinator.
- **Did some of the interviewers respond negatively to your answers?** Try to assess whether it was the content of your response or the tone in which it was delivered. Did you criticize other programs? Did you use a derogatory term to describe a patient? Do your answers sound too rehearsed? Were you overly confident? Did you overemphasize your role in a research project? Ask the opinion of a trusted friend and make adjustments accordingly in your interview approach.
- **Did you not have "any more questions" when asked?** Always ask more questions, even if they have already been asked and answered, or risk sounding disinterested.
- **Were you unprepared to discuss prior research or work experiences in detail?** Review your curriculum vitae (CV) and publications thoroughly. Be ready to intelligently discuss any aspect, from the structure of the study to the basic science behind the work.

If a review of your performance makes you realize that you forgot to mention something of importance, such as a personal tie to the area, consider addressing it in a follow-up communication. However, if the oversight was a blunder on your part, avoid the topic. The program may review any post-interview communication prior to final ranking, so there is no need to remind them that you were late.

Post-Interview Correspondence

Thank You Notes

Within a week of an interview, send a thank you note or email to everyone with whom you interviewed. Many students do this the same day as the interview, while details are fresh in their mind. Thank the interviewers for their time and state that you enjoyed your day, possibly mentioning the most intriguing aspects of the program. Try to personalize the email based on some of the points discussed in your interview. Declaring in a thank you note that the program is your top choice is premature, but if you have geographical or family constraint, it cannot hurt to emphasize them.

Insider Tip: Write a thank you note or email to everyone with whom you interviewed, including Program Directors and Program Coordinators. Either form of communication is fine. Nevertheless, be aware that while an email allows for easy response, do not be upset if you do not receive one.

Unethical Communication

While contact between applicants and programs following the interview is discouraged, it is actually fairly common. In a 2010 study of Emergency Medicine residency applicants, 89% reported some form of post-interview contact, mostly via email (91%), though 55% also reported phone contact [1]. Some programs are subtle, inquiring if you enjoyed your experience or have any additional questions. Others are more blatant, asking an applicant how they will rank their program or, in turn, (falsely) promising a matchable rank position in hopes of improving recruitment. The National Resident Matching Program (NRMP®) strives to maintain the highest level of professionalism throughout the Match process and defines the following as unacceptable post-interview contact [2]:

> Program directors shall not solicit or require post-interview communication from applicants, nor shall program directors engage in post-interview communication that is disingenuous for the purpose of influencing applicants' ranking preferences.

> Program directors and other interviewers may freely express their interest in a candidate, but they shall not require an applicant to disclose ranking preferences, ranking intentions, or the locations of other programs to which the applicant has or may apply.

In a 2000 survey of surgical residency Program Directors asking how post-interview communication with applicants was conducted and interpreted, 47% of programs told students to keep in touch in order to be ranked in a position to match [3]. However, despite this number, 77% of Program Directors said that these affirmations had no effect on students' rank. Moreover, 90% of Program Directors believed that students sometimes lied to them. Clearly, there is an element of gamesmanship in post-interview communications.

Second Looks

There are differing opinions on the value of a second-look visit, and you should tailor your perspective to your own situation. A second-look visit can express interest in a program and answer any questions remaining after interview day. However, if you have already had an excellent interview, you risk detracting from that performance. A second-look visit is generally spent simply shadowing a resident or attending, and keeping up a façade of unflinching interest and enthusiasm throughout the day is no easy feat. It will essentially be an entire day of the dreaded, "Do you have any more questions?" There are also cost considerations. In light of this, the NRMP *Match Communication Code of Conduct* states [4]:

> Program directors shall respect the logistical and financial burden many applicants face in pursuing multiple interactions with programs and shall not require them or imply that second visits are used in determining applicant placement on a rank order list.

Final Contact

At the end of the interview season, in mid to late January, programs begin to prepare their final rank lists. This is the time to reaffirm your interest in a program. These post-season communications carry much more weight than the mandatory post-interview thank you note. While there is no assurance that they will positively affect your rank, they cannot hurt.

If possible, have a faculty member reach out to your top program. From a Program Director perspective, getting a personal call or letter from a trusted and/or respected colleague is always helpful. In some specialties, such as Surgery, it is considered almost essential.

You should also send a "letter of intent." That being said, Program Directors receive a large number of letters containing cryptic statements such as, "You are a top choice" or "You are at the top of my list" and are well-experienced in sorting through the noise. The letter they are really looking for is one that unequivocally states, "I intend to rank your program as number one on my list." Do not be dishonest! The world of residency Program Directors is a small one. Information spreads easily, and lying is not taken lightly. Of course, do not be *too* honest. One of the oddest post-interview letters we ever received stated, "While you are not my top choice, I intend to rank you somewhere between #3 and #5 on my rank list." We decided to spare the candidate the agony of his decision by ranking him lower on our list.

✓ **Insider Tip:** Write an unambiguous "letter of intent" to your top program choice.

Incidentally, do not assume that the lack of a return "We like you, too" letter from the program indicates that you will not be ranked in a position to match. In this case, no news is not necessarily good news, but it certainly is not bad news.

Ranking

Hopefully, our discussion of the matching algorithm in Chapter 1: *The Match Alphabet Soup*, convinced you to form your rank order list (ROL) based on your actual preferences, rather than how you think a program will rank you based on notions of your competitiveness or post-interview promises. Moving a program up your ROL based on these factors alone benefits only the program, not the candidate.

> **Insider Tip:** You have nothing to lose and everything to gain by ranking your favorite program first. You would be doing yourself a huge disservice by structuring your ROL in order to "match at the top of your rank list" if that program was not actually your top choice.

To avoid getting lost in the confusion, revisit the secondary criteria application list you made and have updated throughout the interview season. Review the program-specific comments next to each criterion and, with the knowledge you have gained, reprioritize the criteria if necessary. Then simply rank your list in the order of the programs that satisfy the most of your top-weighted criteria. This is relatively easy if you have been able to articulate on your spreadsheet the facts and feel of the programs. If not, do not underestimate the value of intuition. If you just "liked" one program more without knowing quite sure why, and it does not have major deficits among your essential criteria, then simply rank it higher. Do not overanalyze to the point of paralysis.

> **Insider Tip:** Do not overthink your rank list.

Be sure to rank all the programs that you are willing to attend, including several safety programs at the bottom of your list. The 2013 NRMP *Applicant Survey* revealed that US Seniors who matched ranked an average of 11 programs, while unmatched applicants ranked only six programs [5]. Only leave a program off your list if, after interviewing, you would rather be jobless than attend that program. Remember that the NRMP considers the match participation agreement a binding contract, which can only be nullified by "extreme hardship."

For those applying to advanced positions, you also have to submit a supplemental ROL. To clarify the more common points of confusion on this topic, the NRMP matching algorithm treats these as two separate but sequential lists. In other words, *only* after successfully matching in an advanced PGY-2 position will the system turn to your supplemental list and try to match you in a PGY-1 position. If you fail to match at one of the advanced programs, it will *not* begin to go down your supplemental rank list to ensure that you at least have a PGY-1 position. If you do match in an advanced position, the algorithm simply goes down your supplemental list in order, like your primary ROL. There is no system in place to pair your advanced program with a preliminary program, meaning there is no way to stipulate "If I match in advanced program A, I only want to match in preliminary programs #1–3 (because they are in the same city)."

You do have a few options to consider for your primary ROL. First, you may go the traditional route of maintaining two pure and separate lists, with only advanced positions on your primary list and preliminary positions on your supplemental list. However, with this method you will be completely unmatched if you do not get an advanced position. Alternatively, you can mix your primary ROL. After ranking all your advanced positions on your primary ROL, you can include a few preliminary or transitional year PGY-1 programs. The Match algorithm is neither aware of, nor adjusts in any way for, a change in program or specialty type. Consequently, if rank positions #1–10 are advanced positions and #11–15 are preliminary positions, and you do not match at advanced programs by #10, the system simply moves to #11, a preliminary program. If you successfully match there, your Monday match week message from the NRMP (before detailed results are posted on Friday) will state:

Congratulations, you have matched to a one-year position!

Despite matching at a program from your primary rank list, the NRMP recognizes that this is not a "full" match and rather a "partial" match. Therefore, you are still eligible for the Supplemental Offer and Acceptance Program (SOAP®) for the remainder of your training (SOAP will be discussed extensively in Chapter 12: *Match Week*). By placing a PGY-1 position on your primary rank list, you now only have to scramble for the advanced position, rather than both. If during the interview process you have concluded that you may not be competitive enough for your preferred specialty, and therefore also applied to other specialties or categorical programs, you have a second option. Again, the algorithm permits you to mix specialties and program types on your ROL. Thus, if you would prefer to match in another specialty rather than risk the SOAP, you could rank your list as follows:

1. Advanced Program A (Anesthesiology)
2. Advanced Program B (Anesthesiology)
3. Advanced Program C (Anesthesiology)
4. Categorical Program X (Surgery)
5. Categorical Program Y (Surgery)
6. Categorical Program X (Surgery)
7. Preliminary Program L
8. Preliminary Program M
9. Transitional Program N
10. Preliminary Program O

Insider Tip: If trying to match to an advanced program, consider placing preliminary (PGY-1) programs on your primary ROL. That way you only have to get one residency program, rather than two, through SOAP.

Insider Tip: More details about SOAP are discussed in the next chapter. For now, if you are a high-risk applicant, remember that if you do not match, you may have to apply to another specialty through SOAP. Consider writing an additional personal statement and/or acquiring new LoRs for that backup specialty. There are only 2 hours between notification of "no match" and SOAP application.

For those ranking as a couple, you have to build a much longer rank list than the typical single candidate. Review the section on the Match algorithm in Chapter 1: *The Match Alphabet Soup* to understand the complexities of couples matching. If one of the applicants matching as a couple is a very strong candidate in a less-competitive field, that candidate should consider ranking a "No match" option at the end of their paired ROL. This essentially allows the less-competitive applicant to attempt to match as a single candidate for that iteration. The hope is that the stronger candidate will be able to find a position through SOAP. This is a logical, but scary tactic and only to be placed on your ROL when *all* other viable paired options have been listed first.

Insider Tip: After failing to match as a couple, the NRMP does NOT then re-evaluate each member's rank list as an individual. Thus, it is wise for the stronger applicant to add a few "No match" combinations at the end of the ROL and hope that the unmatched applicant gets a spot through SOAP.

Finally, prepare your ROL with plenty of time to spare and make sure to certify it! The NRMP website (www.nrmp.org) warns that servers may be overloaded and work very slowly at the ROL submission deadline. You will receive a confirmatory email and your user status will switch to "certified." After certification, changes can still be made to your rank list, but you will need to re-certify the list in order to save those changes. The NRMP does *not* store prior versions of your ROL, even certified ones. As far as the NRMP is concerned, the version of your ROL visible on the Registration, Ranking, and Results (R3®) system at login is the *only* version in existence.

Insider Tip: Do *not* be caught without a certified ROL at submission deadline! Certify your ROL with plenty of time to spare.

References

1. Yarris, L. M., Deiorio, N. M., and Gaines, S. S. (2010) Emergency medicine residency applicants' perceptions about being contacted after interview day. *Western Journal of Emergency Medicine* **11** (5): 474–478.

2. NRMP (2012) *Data Release and Research Committee. Results of the 2012 NRMP Program Director Survey.* Washington, DC: National Resident Matching Program.

3. Anderson, K. D. and Jacobs, D. M. (2000) General surgery program directors' perceptions of the match. *Current Surgery* **57** (5): 460–465.

4. NRMP. Match Communication Code of Conduct; available from: http://www.nrmp.org/code-of-conduct/ [accessed September 2014].

5. NRMP (2013) *Data Release and Research Committee: Results of the 2013 NRMP Applicant Survey by Preferred Specialty and Applicant Type.* Washington, DC: National Resident Matching Program.

Chapter 11

12: Match Week

Congratulations, it's here! You are so close you can taste it (or maybe that is your stress-induced acid reflux). All the hard work and anxiety of the last few years are about to pay off. Students have varied responses to Match Week. Some of the more confident applicants look forward to the Match Week festivities with excitement. Others who are fearful of embarrassment or disappointment disappear. They would rather find out the Match results online in the privacy of their own home or favorite vacation spot rather than in-person for their whole school to see. But as nerve-racking as it is, we recommend that you stay local, if not on-site. First, everyone's Match results are posted online at the exact same moment. This can be a strain on bandwidth capabilities, so you may have to go to your happy place and practice deep-breathing exercises while you await access to the site. Second, and more importantly, on the slim chance you do not get a residency spot, if on-site, you can immediately begin working with your Dean's Office to make preparations for the Supplemental Offer and Acceptance Program (SOAP®). The National Resident Matching Program (NRMP®) website (www.nrmp.org) discusses in detail the current year's Match Week schedule, but the following is a basic overview. More comprehensive information regarding the SOAP schedule is explained in the next section. **All times discussed in this chapter are in Eastern Standard Time (ET).**

Friday (prior to Match Week)	All SOAP-eligible applicants are notified of their eligibility. Do not panic! This is in no way reflective of whether or not you matched.
Monday 12 p.m. (noon)	Program Directors find out if they filled all their residency positions. Applicants learn if they matched completely or partially, or are unmatched. <ul><li>Note that it is possible to match to an advanced position on your primary rank order list (ROL), but not match into a preliminary position on your supplemental ROL. If that is the case, you are still under the NRMP's binding agreement to attend the advanced program. Your options are to pursue a PGY-1 position either through SOAP as part of the Match or by contacting unfilled programs after Match Week has concluded. The latter is much riskier, as the vast majority of positions will fill through SOAP.</li><li>If SOAP-eligible and fully or partially unmatched, you will have access to a list of unfilled programs on the NRMP website at this time.</li></ul>
Monday 1 p.m.	SOAP-eligible applicants begin applying to available residency positions through Electronic Residency Application Service (ERAS®) (available for program download at 2 p.m.). Through a series of rounds, residency positions are offered and accepted or rejected by applicants.
Thursday 5 p.m.	SOAP closes.
Friday 1 p.m.	Match results are posted in NRMP Registration, Ranking, and Results (R3®) system.

Be sure to check the NRMP website to validate the timeline for your application cycle.

SOAP

Due to the combined efforts of the Association of American Medical Colleges (AAMC) and the NRMP, SOAP was introduced in 2012 under the stewardship of the NRMP in order to replace the chaotic and decentralized 2-day scramble. Previously, the scramble began 1 day after applicants were notified that they did not match. Applicants often recruited friends, family, or even companies to participate in a massive campaign the following day by submitting ERAS applications while simultaneously calling and faxing programs directly. In 2010, the number of applicants participating in the scramble had swelled to 13 000 applicants; combined with these frantic campaigns, it was utter pandemonium. Programs were desperate to pull their spots from the calling pool as quickly as possible, so that landing a vacant position was very much a matter of first come, first served. With SOAP, the process is much more streamlined and less frenzied. The planning day has been eliminated, as applicants are only given 2 hours notification between learning that they did not match and submitting their updated applications into ERAS, now the singular means of application. Applicants are strictly prohibited from initiating contact with the programs. Once a program downloads an application, if interested they will reach out to the student and conduct an interview either via phone or Skype.

SOAP Eligibility

Participation in SOAP is considered part of the Match and falls under its binding commitment. Therefore, on the Friday before Match Week, NRMP ensures that *all* applicants are still eligible by requiring medical schools and the Educational Commission for Foreign Medical Graduates (ECFMG®) to re-certify applicant status. According to the NRMP website, in order to be considered "verified," an applicant must be:

1. Registered for the NRMP Main Residency Match® (deadline is mid to late February)
2. Fully or partially unmatched
3. Eligible to enter residency training on July 1 in the year of the Match

A few points of clarification on SOAP eligibility:

- Registration for the NRMP Match is in no way related to either your ROL or your ERAS application. If you decided after the application deadlines to change specialties and thus did not actually apply to any programs, or if you applied but received no interviews, or if you were planning on using SOAP as your primary means of application, you are eligible. You are not required to have submitted applications nor ranked programs in order to participate in SOAP. We do, however, recommend that you have a viable application on file with MyERAS so it is ready to go for SOAP. You can even consider sending it to a program, no matter how unlikely your chances of consideration, to make sure there are no technical glitches in the download of your application. If you have already applied to programs through ERAS, there are no additional fees for SOAP.

- If you are fully unmatched, you have to consider applying to either categorical positions or again to both preliminary and advanced positions. If you are partially unmatched, you can only re-apply to the missing part of your training. This means that if you matched for an advanced position in Boston but do not want to move twice, you cannot disregard that match and start all over again in a different city. When it comes to SOAP, "take what you can get" and just deal with whatever issues may arise from moving.
- To be considered eligible for entering into training on July 1, US medical schools must re-certify that their seniors are on track to graduate on time. ECFMG will verify that International Medical Graduates (IMGs) have passed their required examinations (United States Medical Licensing Examination® (USMLE®) Levels 1, 2 CK (Clinical Knowledge) and 2 CS (Clinical Skills)). A common point of confusion is that IMGs often think that their ECFMG certification status must be "complete" before they can participate in the Match (including SOAP), which would mean that they must have already graduated medical school. This is not the case, you must simply be on track to graduate by July 1 [1].

In 2013, there were 1041 first- and second-year positions unfilled after the conclusion of the matching algorithm, with 13 808 SOAP-eligible applicants vying for these positions. Non-US citizen IMGs constituted the greater part (44%), followed by US citizen IMGs (27%), US Seniors (15%), and osteopathic medical school graduates (7%). However, despite these numbers, US Seniors took the majority of positions (68%) filled during SOAP [2]. It is this discrepancy that worries IMGs, as many feel that in the turmoil of the first-come, first-served scramble, there was a more level playing field. Unlike the previous system, SOAP allows programs to see the entire applicant pool all at once and potentially filter by citizenship status. NRMP Match data results prior to the institution of SOAP did not differentiate whether matched IMGs obtained residency positions as part of the matching algorithm or in the scramble. Therefore, it is difficult to draw an objective comparison between an IMG's chances to secure a position in the old versus the new system. Nevertheless, it would seem reasonable for IMGs to be concerned.

SOAP Logistics and Schedule

Unfilled residency programs choosing to participate in the Match use the NRMP's web-based R3 system and a preference list to offer positions to SOAP-eligible unmatched applicants through a series of rounds. A program's participation in SOAP is optional and they may elect to fill their positions outside the Match. However, once having agreed to participate in the Match, they cannot pursue this route until Match Week has concluded. In 2013, 406 (85%) of the 476 unfilled programs chose to participate in SOAP, offering 939 (90%) of the 1041 positions not filled at the completion of the matching algorithm [2]. Of these, just over half (57.6%) were PGY-1 only, predominantly preliminary positions in Surgery (Figure 12.1). Other substantial minorities included Family Medicine (123 spots), Anesthesiology (31 categorical and 13 advanced), and Diagnostic Radiology (13 categorical and 46 advanced) [2].

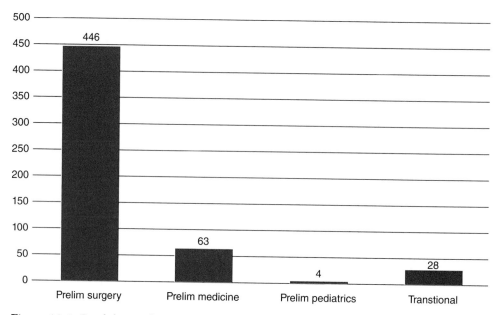

Figure 12.1 Breakdown of PGY-1-only positions offered in the 2013 SOAP. *Source*: Adapted with permission from [2].

The list of available unfilled positions is posted at the same time that students learn that they have not matched – noon on Monday of Match Week. Students should immediately go to their school's predetermined "war room," usually the office of a Dean or advisor, to strategize and ensure that a recent transcript has been uploaded. One hour later (1 p.m.), ERAS opens in SOAP mode so that applicants can begin organizing their application by assigning documents to selected programs. New LoRs and personal statements also can be uploaded, but the short time frame will likely not permit this unless you have prepared them ahead of time. You will be allowed to apply to a maximum of 45 programs, 35 in the first cycle, and 10 in the second cycle. You may re-apply to programs you applied to during the regular Match, regardless of whether or not they interviewed you. If you did not get a spot at any of them prior to SOAP, it means they did not rank you. However, given the situation, they now may view your application in a different light. Note that at this stage only the programs express preferences about the applicants to be selected, based on the assumption that you will happily attend any program that accepts you. In other words, applicants do not create a rank or preference list in NRMP, while residency programs do.

 Insider Tip: While some sources indicate the contrary, as of 2014, applicants do not create a ROL as part of SOAP. Preference is indicated by application alone. However, programs *can* submit a preference list.

Two hours after notification (2 p.m.), residency programs can begin downloading your material. Throughout the remainder of Monday, all of Tuesday, and Wednesday morning, programs will review your application materials. You can track who has downloaded your application through the Applicant Document Tracking System (ADTS) on ERAS. If a program is interested in your application, they will contact you (not the other way around). They may call for an interview or arrange one via email. You must stay in constant contact during this time. There are no "hours of operation" on these communications and you may receive phone calls late into the evening. Be cognizant of time zone differences. If you are scheduled for clinical duties, get out of them. Your clerkships will understand the gravity of the situation and undoubtedly release you from service.

> **Insider Tip:** You *must* be available by phone and email during both the application review and offer phases of SOAP. Some programs will receive hundreds of applications for each vacancy. Given time constraints, not answering your phone for an interview is reason enough for a Program Director to move on to the next applicant.

During the offer rounds, vacant spots in a residency program will be offered to applicants in order of preference until the position is filled or the list is exhausted (the list can be updated once, before the first round). In each round, an applicant has 2 hours to accept or reject the offer or it will expire. Acceptance automatically generates a digital commitment and the position is removed from the list of those unfilled.

> **Insider Tip:** Once an offer is accepted, it is removed from the Unfilled Position List. This list is updated in real time for Program Directors, but not for applicants. The updated list is made available to the applicants after the first round is completed.

If an offer is rejected or expires, it is presented to the next applicant on the list during the next round. If a program has two unfilled positions, they can make a maximum of two offers per round. However, an applicant may receive multiple offers per round. We strongly suggest that you take an offer in the earliest round possible. Do not pass up an offer hoping that your dream program will make an offer in the next one. In the 2012 SOAP, 87% of vacant positions were filled by the end of the second round on the first day (Figure 12.2) [3]. During that first year of SOAP, there were 3 days of round offers. However, when it was shown that less than 1% of positions were filled on the third and final day, SOAP was reduced to 2 days of offers (Wednesday and Thursday).

> **Insider Tip:** Take an offer in the earliest round you can.

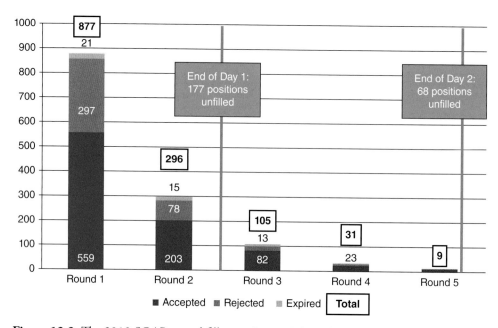

Figure 12.2 The 2012 SOAP round fill rate. *Source:* Adapted with permission from [3].

Due to the newness of the program and the recent structural changes, the schedule for SOAP is a bit confusing and there is a surprising amount of inaccurate information on the web. Below is the SOAP schedule (adapted from the NRMP and ERAS websites) [4, 5] which is accurate at the time of publication in 2014. Be sure to validate the times for your application cycle online.

Monday (Match Week) 12 p.m. (noon)	Applicants finds out they did not match. SOAP-eligible applicants can view the Unfilled Program List through the NRMP's R3 system.

Insider Tip: If you did not match and will participate in SOAP, go immediately to your school's previously designated SOAP location with your laptop, binder of application materials, and cell phone. You will need to discuss options with your advisor and likely have to make some tough geographic decisions that may need input from loved ones.

1 p.m.	ERAS opens for SOAP-eligible applicants. Update your application and begin assigning documents to programs listed as "Unfilled" on the NRMP website.

Insider Tip: Given the high fill rate on the first day, submit applications to the maximum allowed number of programs as soon as possible, preferably before programs begin to download applications. Programs will receive hundreds of applications per position and are unlikely to download any more after a certain point. Also, there likely will be little change between the preference lists they establish based on this cycle of applications versus the next.

Insider Tip: Be flexible in your criteria regarding location and specialty. As the saying goes, "Beggars can't be choosers."

2 p.m.	Programs begin downloading applications. You can check the status of downloads on ADTS. From this point through the first round of offers, programs will review applications and reach out for an interview if interested.

Insider Tip: In this agonizing time period, research the programs to which you applied. Should you get an interview, be ready to give a few reasons why you would want to go there. With the applicant-to-position ratio stacked in favor of the programs, they can afford to choose the most qualified applicant who actually *wants* to go there.

Insider Tip: You may be lucky and receive multiple offers in the first round. With only a 2-hour time period to accept or reject the offer, now is the time to make a mental or unofficial preference list of the programs to which you applied.

Tuesday **11:30 am**	Programs can begin submitting preference lists.
Wednesday *Round 1* **11:55 a.m.** **12 p.m. (noon)–** **2 p.m.**	Program preference list certification deadline for first round. Electronic offers extended to applicants using R3 system in order of preference. Number of program offers extended per round is limited by the number of vacancies. Offers must be accepted or rejected in these 2 hours or they will expire. Once an offer has been made to an applicant and not accepted, programs cannot again offer that applicant a position in a later round.

Insider Tip: Begin *readying* your list for the next 10 applications available for download for Rounds 2–5. Make a list much longer than 10, as many of these will be filled when the Unfilled Position list is updated for applicant viewing shortly after the end of the first round. You need to be able to act quickly. If you submit applications before reviewing this list, many of these 10 will be wasted on positions filled during Round 1.

2:30 p.m.	Apply to remaining 10 programs. You will be able to add these through 5 p.m. on Thursday, but the earlier the better.

Insider Tip: Your initial 35 applications will carry over to subsequent rounds. No need to worry about trying to re-apply to them for the next cycle.

Round 2	
2:55 p.m.	Deadline for programs to add to and certify preference list for next round.
3–5 p.m.	Electronic offers extended.

Insider Tip: While at this point, programs can technically begin downloading the additional 10 applications you submitted, given the short time between Rounds 1 and 2, programs will not realistically have had a chance to review these end applications and likely just go down the same preference list they established before Round 1.

Thursday	
Round 3	
9–11 a.m.	Offers extended electronically.
Round 4	
12–2 p.m.	Offers extended electronically.
Round 5	
3–5 p.m.	Offers extended electronically. SOAP closes at 5 p.m.

Friday	
12 p.m. (noon)	Match Day ceremonies.
1 p.m.	Applicants find out where they matched by email or the R3 system.

Insider Tip: SOAP is still part of the Match. If you received an offer by the close of SOAP at 5 p.m. on Thursday, feel free to participate in your school's Match Day Ceremony. You earned it!

References

1. ECFMG: Ask The Experts – NRMP's SOAP; available from: http://www.ecfmg.org/echo/experts-nrmp-soap.html [accessed March 2014].

2. NRMP (2013) *Results and Data: 2013 Main Residency Match*®. Washington, DC: National Resident Matching Program.

3. Signer, M. (2013) *Main Residency Match: NRMP Update [to the AAMC]. 2014.* Washington, DC: National Resident Matching Program.

4. 2014 Main Residency Match: Match Week and SOAP Schedule; available from: http://b83c73bcf0e7ca356c80-e8560f466940e4ec38ed51af32994bc6.r6.cf1.rackcdn.com/wp-content/uploads/2014/01/2014-Match-Week-Schedule.pdf [accessed March 2014].

5. SOAP 2014: ERAS Applicant Checklist; available from: https://www.aamc.org/download/273512/data/soap_check_students.pdf [accessed March 2014].

Chapter 12

13: International Medical Graduate Specifics

Kenneth B. Christopher, MD
Brigham and Women's Hospital, Harvard Medical School, Boston, MA

Introduction

International Medical Graduates (IMGs) have been training in the United States for decades and have represented up to 30% of the hospital residency workforce in this country. Thousands of physicians who attended medical school from all over the world now practice clinically in the United States, although some IMG physicians who train in the United States return home, bringing unique expertise and perspectives back to their countries. The application process for residency in the United States for IMGs is somewhat similar to that of US Seniors. However, the application strategy is very different, with heavy emphasis placed on United States Medical Licensing Examination® (USMLE®) Step 1 scores and prior clinical experience in the United States.

It must be noted that the landscape for IMG applicants is changing. Attaining a residency spot in the United States for an IMG is becoming much more difficult. In an effort to avoid future physician shortages driven by an aging US population, the Association of American Medical Colleges (AAMC) in 2006 called for an increase in medical school enrollment by 30%. In response, four new medical schools were established and 10% of US medical schools increased enrollment by at least 10%. First-year class sizes have increased more than 20% since 2002. This growth of medical school enrollment, without an increase in federal graduate medical education funding, has put a squeeze on IMGs seeking residency spots. As US medical schools have steadily increased enrollment, the percentage of hospital residency spots taken by IMGs in the United States has declined. This has resulted in a much more competitive process, with IMG candidates who would have matched in a residency in prior years not currently matching.

For those who are interested in coming to the United States to train, it is first important to realize that the odds are stacked against you. According to 2013 figures from the National Resident Matching Program (NRMP®) [1], of those who participated in the Main Residency Match®, interviewed for residency, and submitted certified rank order lists, 22% were non-US IMGs and 15% were US IMGs (those IMGs with US citizenship or permanent resident status). Of those who interviewed for residency, 48% of US IMGs matched and 44% of non-US IMGs matched. It must be noted that when one includes all applicants to residency, including the substantial proportion who do not interview, the percentage of all IMG applicants who actually match into a residency position was approximately 25%.

In general, IMG applicants who do match have robust USMLE Step 1 scores, do not fail any USMLE Step (including the clinical skills exam), are recent graduates, and have clinical experience in the United States [1]. Those who are considered US IMGs, especially those with

US citizenship who speak English as a first language, have an advantage over non-US IMGs with regard to attaining a residency match [1].

USMLE Scores

It is impossible to overemphasize the importance of high USMLE scores. For most IMG candidates, the USMLE scores are the only variable that they can control. Many candidates make the mistake of rushing their preparation to apply quickly following medical school graduation, thinking that programs favor the most recent graduates. While it is true that most IMGs who match graduate near the match date, a recent graduation date cannot make up for poor USMLE scores or having to make more than one attempt to pass an exam required for Educational Commission for Foreign Medical Graduates (ECFMG®) certification. According to the NRMP, the mean (± standard deviation) USMLE Step 1 score among US IMG applicants who match is 217 ± 18 and for non-US IMG applicants is 227 ± 19 [1]. However, certain specialty-specific training programs require scores well above the mean to even be granted an interview and possibly match. Five percent of those who take the clinical skills exam fail and nearly all are IMGs. Many IMGs underestimate the difficulty of the clinical skills exam and the serious consequences of failing.

For an IMG, exam preparation should take precedence over all other activities. A few weeks of preparation and study will not suffice. Those who are successful in matching spend a large amount of time on exam preparation, typically 6 months to 2 years. Since a 2-year gap between completion of medical school and one's application is not desirable, consider studying for the USMLE during medical school to reduce the amount of time needed to prepare after graduation. At its core, the exam is about concepts rather than random facts. Exam preparation needs to be mapped out and it takes much more time than one would expect. For example, deeply reading and retaining a high-yield review book can take 10 days. *First Aid for the USMLE Step 1* [2], should be reviewed multiple times. Furthermore, a 2000-item question bank can take up to 200 hours to finish and many more than this number of questions is required to be adequately prepared. Question banks should be done in random order and timed. Trying to guess the answer to the question before looking at the options will improve retention of concepts.

Question banks should be considered as learning tools rather than for their assessment value and question banks from at least two sources should be completed. Answering questions is a form of active learning, which should take precedence over reading text to memorize information. Working through a large number of questions also helps one learn the art of making intelligent guesses. It is essential that one utilize the National Board of Medical Examiners (NBME) questions as a learning and assessment tool. Concepts tested on the NBME questions are very frequently seen on the USMLE Step 1 and these questions are a reliable assessment tool to determine whether you are ready to take the exam. It is important to complete at the very least two NBME practice tests prior to the exam and not take USMLE Step 1 if the scores are poor. Many people underestimate the difficulty of the exam and the time it takes to get the score one needs to match.

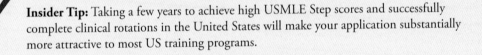

Insider Tip: Set aside sufficient time to prepare for the USMLE Step exams, because a high score is critical to maximize your chance of matching into a residency program.

Recent Graduates

In general, IMGs who match do so within 5 years of graduation. Many programs in Internal Medicine indicate on their websites that IMGs must have graduated within 5 years, though this is not a legal requirement and there are exceptions. Nevertheless, in Internal Medicine, the mean number of years following graduation among those who match is 1.7 years for US IMGs and 4.3 years for non-US IMG applicants [1]. The situation is similar in Family Medicine, with a mean time since graduation of 1.7 years among US IMGs and 3.6 years for non-US IMG applicants [1]. In general, IMGs who do not match in Internal Medicine or Family Medicine have graduated more than 5 years prior to applying. The underlying message is that most IMG candidates who successfully match do not match straight out of medical school.

Insider Tip: Taking a few years to achieve high USMLE Step scores and successfully complete clinical rotations in the United States will make your application substantially more attractive to most US training programs.

Clinical Experience in the United States

Clinical experience in the United States is a very important part of an application for an IMG, especially as the Medical Student Performance Evaluation (MSPE) from many international schools is non-existent or not comparable to those coming from US schools. In addition, most Program Directors have no easy way to assess the meaning of grades from foreign schools, since they have no idea of their academic status. The most valuable US clinical experience is as a medical student, where you are able to examine and manage patients as part of a care team. Of major importance, this enables you to be evaluated as a student by US physicians in an academic medical center, who will likely be happy to write a letter in support of your residency application. US clinical experience as a student is far more valuable than an observership after graduating from medical school, in which your interactions with patients are minimal, or a clinical experience in the office of a private physician, where your activities may constitute the illegal practice of medicine without a license if they exceed those routinely fulfilled by a medical assistant [3]. A rotation (also known as a clerkship) as a medical student is a true "hands-on" experience and your evaluations or letters of reference can comment on your clinical management as well as physical examination skills. These clinical experiences also permit an assessment of your communication and interpersonal skills. Program Directors worry about how well foreign medical students possess these critical abilities and successful completion of a clinical rotation in the United States helps to decrease these concerns.

US IMGs who study in Caribbean medical schools have the opportunity to complete rotations as medical students in hospitals in the United States. Non-US IMGs are able to do rotations as medical students in the United States if their own institutions allow such rotations and if the students plan far enough in advance. Some medical schools outside the United States have agreements with US medical schools for student exchanges. Some students from outside the United States do rotations in the United States as students after completing medical school, but before their diplomas are granted. It is best to do these rotations while as student in your final year, as you will be expected to function with some independence. The AAMC provides an online list of medical schools that are willing to host students from a medical schools outside the United States [4]. Students need to be proactive about securing these types of clinical experiences early, as the process may be competitive and costly.

> **Insider Tip:** Clinical experience in the United States is an essential part of any residency application, as it allows for first-hand assessment of the clinical knowledge and communication and interpersonal skills of an IMG.

Research Fellowships and/or Graduate Degrees

For physicians, pursuing research fellowships or even a Masters degree in a field that one is passionately interested in may be helpful. However, graduate degrees (MPH, PhD) completed in the United States are not designed to improve your residency application. Occasionally, obtaining an additional degree, such as a Masters in a clinical science field at a strong program, followed by a time working as a productive clinical researcher, can be the difference between matching and not matching. The downside is that Masters programs are expensive and many research fellowships come with no or minimal salary. The time and money required to attain a Masters degree is best spent after completing residency training.

Some IMGs spend 1–2 years as a research fellow in the United States. This tactic has several advantages, not the least of which is that it allows one the opportunity to build personal relationships with US physicians. Sometimes, this can lead to residency opportunities in the hospital in which one is working. If you do decide to pursue a research fellowship, it is important to select the right Principal Investigator. Do not jump at the first opportunity available. Perform due diligence and determine whether or not the hospital and department in which you will be working has ever accepted an IMG researcher as a resident. Some prestigious institutions may not even consider IMGs for residency spots even after they have researched there. Generally, it is best to work for a senior member of the field, but make sure you research their track record of placing research fellows in residency spots. When working for some highly regarded physicians, you may be one of multiple research fellows and it will be difficult to stand out. If you do decide to pursue a research fellowship, it is important that you do an outstanding job and be productive! An absence of publications and lack of a letter of recommendation from you research mentor are "red flags."

It must be stressed that research fellowships or a Masters degree are not substitutes for poor USMLE scores or a USMLE failure.

> **Insider Tip:** Although pursuing research or even a Masters degree is one possible path to strengthening your application, do not count on getting into residency based solely upon this one aspect of your application.

What Field and Where to Apply

It is critical to be realistic about what field and where to apply. No residency is impossible to get into, as even the best programs in the country recognize that talent has no borders. Nevertheless, it is most likely that an IMG will match at a program that historically accepts IMGs. Some websites (e.g., Internal Medicine Residency for IMGs; im-for-imgs.com) provide tables listing IMG friendly programs. Another source of information is seeing which US programs have matched graduates from your own medical school. A residency program with a positive experience in training graduates from a specific medical school in the past is much more apt to take other qualified applicants from the same school. A good example of this type of relationship is Henry Ford Hospital, which has matched a number of IMGs from Universidad Peruana Cayetano Heredia in Lima, Peru.

The field to which one applies is also important. The majority of IMGs match in Internal Medicine. Family Medicine may have lower mean USMLE scores, but overall there are fewer residency spots available. Of the 6612 first-year residency spots in Internal Medicine, 841 (13%) were filled by US IMG applicants and 1690 (26%) by non-US IMG applicants [1]. For Family Medicine, there were 3037 first-year residency spots, of which 531 (17%) were filled by US IMG applicants and 293 (10%) by non-US IMG applicants [1]. Of the 1362 first-year residency spots in Psychiatry, 15% were filled by US IMGs and 12% were filled by non-US IMGs [1]. In contrast, some fields are very difficult to match to as an IMG. For example, of the 116 first-year Plastic Surgery residency spots offered, only two (2%) were filled by non-US IMG applicants and none were filled by US IMGs. Table 13.1 lists those specialties with 100 or more IMG applicants.

> **Insider Tip:** Both the field and the program to which one applies can impact the chances of an IMG of attaining a residency position in a US program. Some fields and programs are more competitive, whereas others are more receptive to training IMGs.

Chapter 13

Table 13.1 Specialties with a high number of IMG applicants

Specialty	Total positions	US IMG		Non-US IMG	
		Matched	No match	Matched	No match
Anesthesiology	1653	95	65	78	85
Emergency Medicine	1744	53	137	31	53
Family Medicine	3037	531	702	293	616
General Surgery	1185	119	123	158	150
Internal Medicine	6612	841	753	1690	1856
Neurology	692	59	44	148	149
Obstetrics and Gynecology	1237	78	99	62	120
Pathology	583	46	69	151	136
Pediatrics	2699	196	151	278	382
Physical Medicine and Rehabilitation	397	40	43	21	26
Psychiatry	1362	203	256	163	277
Radiology	1143	55	47	66	63

Source: Data adapted with permission from the NRMP based upon the 2014 Main Residency Match.

Application

The ECFMG was established in 1956 to assess and certify IMGs for medical training in the United States. In order to apply to an ACGME accredited program, one must obtain ECFMG certification. This ensures that IMGs have met minimum standards before entrusting them with patient care. Between 1986 and 2005, of more than 267 000 IMGs undergoing the certification process, only 57.2% were ultimately successful [5]. To be eligible for certification, an IMG must meet the following requirements:

Application for ECFMG certification	Complete an application confirming identity, contact information, and graduation/enrollment in a medical school listed in the *International Medical Education Directory (IMED)*
Examination requirements	Pass USMLE Steps 1, 2 CK (Clinical Knowledge) and 2 CS (Clinical Skills)
Education requirements	Be a graduate of a medical school listed in the *IMED*
	Be awarded credit for at least 4 academic years
	Document completion of all requirements for, and receipt of, a medical diploma
	Provide a medical transcript

The ECFMG then performs a rigorous primary-source verification process. This ensures that IMGs have met minimum standards. Make sure to visit the ECFMG website (www.ecfmg.org) for full details.

After obtaining ECFMG certification, it is time to turn your attention to the application. Chapter 7: *The Application*, Chapter 8: *The Curriculum Vitae*, and Chapter 9: *The Personal Statement* of this book summarize the application process. The goal is to have the structure of your application as an IMG look like an application from a US medical student. The application should showcase your strengths and what you can bring to the training program. As there are thousands of applicants for a limited number of positions, it is most important that your application is as good as it can be. It should appear that you spent a large amount of time crafting it. You should have a native English speaker review the application for spelling and grammar errors. Running your application through a spell-check program is not sufficient! Your personal statement needs to be original, clear, concise, and not copied from any other sources. It should allow the reader to understand where you came from, what you have done to date, and what you aspire to do in the future. However, keep in mind that anything mentioned in the personal statement and application narratives will be topics for discussion if you are asked to come for an interview. It is imperative that one is honest on the application and not boastful. Manuscripts that are listed as submitted, accepted, or published are easy to check for validity. Any concern of dishonesty or arrogance in your application will not bode well for a successful match. Also, submit a picture with your application where you are smiling (even though the requirements are for a "neutral" expression). A picture with a smile shows that you are friendly and collegial. Make sure that the picture uploads and looks professional. Remember that programs are selecting residents with whom they will work for multiple years; they want people who will be altruistic, provide excellent care to patients, work well with others, and be trustworthy. Finally, make sure you apply broadly to both small and larger programs. Every program receives hundreds to thousands of applications for relatively few positions, so this will maximize your chance of receiving a reasonable number of interviews.

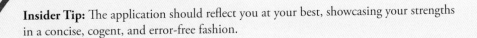

Insider Tip: The application should reflect you at your best, showcasing your strengths in a concise, cogent, and error-free fashion.

Interview

The interview is essential to securing a residency position. The interview is an opportunity to have a conversation with a prospective colleague, and for you to share your interests and future aspirations. Applicants who interview well are able to speak on the topics that they know well (their applications), as well as ask interesting questions of the interviewer. You should have prepared an "elevator talk" – a 2-minute pitch that summarizes why you are interested in the particular field. You should practice this pitch out loud in front of a mirror to get used to saying the words smoothly or in front of a few friends who can provide constructive feedback. Some medical schools provide "mock interviews" for their students and you should strongly consider participating in one of these sessions. Make sure to review the practice questions emphasized in Chapter 10: *The Interview*. It is important to realize that the interview is not scripted and therefore should be a conversation that flows easily. The interviewer expects questions and looks for applicants who ask insightful questions indicating that they have done their homework about the program.

> **Insider Tip:** A good question at the end of the interview, which shows that you have researched the program prior to your visit, will often leave a positive impression in the interviewer's mind.

There are many good questions that can be asked. Some can be as simple as "What keeps you at this institution?" or "What do you like most about your work here?" These will leave you with a sense of what are the most positive aspects of the program or hospital. More complex questions might be along the lines of, "Looking at your website, I was impressed at how many residents are actively pursuing research during their training. I am very interested in research and would be interested in learning more about what specific opportunities exist in your program."

Finally, non-verbal cues during the interview are important. Try not to fold your arms. Lean forward about 5 degrees and be animated when talking about things for which you are passionate. Try to be relaxed and friendly, and do not forget to smile. It is natural to be nervous, but remember that your interviewers are generally trying to get to know you as a person and develop a sense of what it would be like to work with you.

Communication

Following the interview, communication with the program should be kept to a minimum. A simple "Thank you for your time and consideration on interview day" statement in an email will suffice. No candidate is judged on the quality or content of their thank you card or email. There is no expectation of any communication from the candidate by the program. Excessive communication can be construed in a negative way. The exception to this general advice is when an applicant has a new achievement, such as a publication to add to their curriculum vitae (CV). Finally, communication received by the program from mentors who can vouch for you as a candidate can be quite helpful, especially if your mentor happens to know the Program Director or Department Chairman personally.

Visas

Finally, brief mention must be made about visas. IMGs visiting and working in the United States require a visa. A visitor B1/B2 visa allows IMGs to attend interviews in the United States. In order to work in the country, two common types of visas are available to IMGs: J-1 and H-1B visas.

- A **J-1 visa** is sponsored by the ECFMG and is a temporary, non-immigrant visa reserved for educational training purposes. J-1 visas last for the duration of training, up to a maximum of 7 years. Dependents of J-1 visa holders may obtain J-2 visas, which will allow them to work and live legally in the United States. The J-1 visa has several disadvantages, not the least of which is the 2-year home-country physical presence requirement (Section 212(e) of the Immigration and Nationality Act). This provision requires visa holders to return to their home countries for 2 years following their expiration of their visas. Waivers can be obtained for several reasons, including providing medical service to an underserved area in the United States, but usually require the assistance of an immigration lawyer. Another limitation associated with the J-1 visa is that holders may only change their specialty once during the first 2 years of training. After the third year of training, a change in specialty is no longer permitted.

- An **H-1B visa** is sponsored by the trainee's hospital and is a working visa with a duration up to 6 years. Holders of H-1B visas have significant advantages over those with J-1 visas, in that they are not subject to the 2-year home-country physical presence requirement and can apply for permanent residence following visa expiration. Dependents of an H-1B visa are eligible for an H-4 visa, which allows them to stay in the country, but does not allow them to work. Given the advantages of the H-1B visa, one may wonder why all IMGs do not apply for one. First, the number of H-1B visas is capped at 65 000 per year, although there are many exceptions; in 2012, 135 991 were issued. Second, there is considerable paperwork and cost associated with issuance of the H-1B visa, which dissuades many sponsoring institutions from offering them. While all of this may seem like a tremendous hassle, if you are at this stage, you have successfully matched and should be congratulated!

A last piece of advice is to keep your eyes and ears open at all times. Even some of the best programs may have unexpected openings. Some IMGs are fortunate to discover these openings, and submit their letters of interest and CVs directly to the programs, as these positions almost always fall outside of the match. Most of these unexpected openings are listed on a variety of internet sites; some of the most common are www.ama-assn.org, www.residentswap.org, www.inforesidency.com, and www.openresidencypositions.com. In order to maximize your chance of securing one of these openings, having a mentor call the program on your behalf can be particularly helpful.

Chapter 13

References

1. NRMP and ECFMG. Charting Outcomes in the Match for International Medical Graduates; available from: http://www.ecfmg.org/resources/NRMP-ECFMG-Charting-Outcomes-in-the-Match-International-Medical-Graduates-2014.pdf [accessed September 2014].
2. Le, T. and Bhuskan, V. (2014) *First Aid for the USMLE Step 1*. New York, NY: McGraw-Hill Education.
3. Medical Board of California. Warning to physicians and program directors: don't assist the unlicensed practice of medicine; available from: http://www.mbc.ca.gov/publications/newsletters/newsletter_2010_07.pdf [accessed September 2014].
4. AAMC. On-Line Extramural Electives Compendium; available from: https://services.aamc.org/eec/students/index.cfm [accessed September 2014].
5. ECFMG. About ECFMG Certification; available from: http://www.ecfmg.org/certification/index.html [accessed September 2014].

Index